SHUT AWAY

CATHERINE McKERCHER

SHUT AWAY

WHEN **DOWN SYNDROME** WAS A **LIFE SENTENCE**

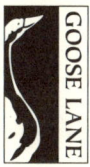

GOOSE LANE

Edited by Jill Ainsley.
Cover and page design by Julie Scriver.
Cover image: "Bill in the park at Smiths Falls," courtesy Catherine McKercher.
All photographs courtesy Catherine McKercher unless otherwise indicated.
Printed in Canada.
10 9 8 7 6 5 4 3 2 1

Library and Archives Canada Cataloguing in Publication

Title: Shut away : when Down syndrome was a life sentence / Catherine McKercher.
Names: McKercher, Catherine, 1952- author.

Description: Includes bibliographical references.
Identifiers: Canadiana (print) 20190090669 | Canadiana (ebook) 20190090782 |
ISBN 9781773100982 (softcover) | ISBN 9781773101002 (EPUB) | ISBN 9781773100999 (Kindle)
Subjects: LCSH: McKercher, Catherine, 1952-—Family. | LCSH: Down syndrome—Patients—
Family relationships. | LCSH: Intellectual disability facilities patients—Abuse of—Canada. |
LCSH: People with mental disabilities—Abuse of—Canada. | LCSH: People with mental
disabilities—Care—Canada. | LCSH: Intellectual disability facilities—Canada. |
LCSH: Mental health facilities—Canada.
Classification: LCC HV3008.C2 M35 2019 | DDC 362.20971—dc23

Goose Lane Editions acknowledges the generous financial support of the Government of Canada, the Canada Council for the Arts, and the Province of New Brunswick.

Goose Lane Editions
500 Beaverbrook Court, Suite 330
Fredericton, New Brunswick
CANADA E3B 5X4
www.gooselane.com

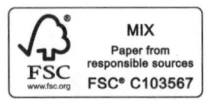

MIX
Paper from
responsible sources
FSC® C103567

For Bill

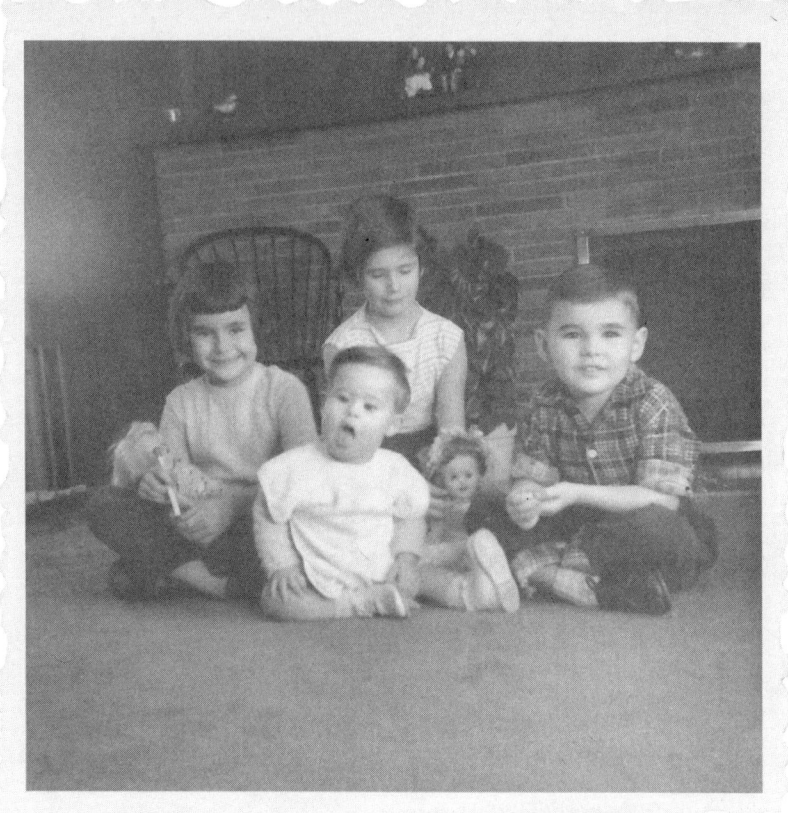

A rare snapshot of all four McKercher children at home in Ottawa.
This was probably the last photo of Bill taken before his move
to the Ontario Hospital School in February of 1959.

Contents

Introduction

"How many brothers and sisters do you have?"

It was one of the first questions kids asked each other back in the 1950s and 1960s, when big families were common. I never knew how to answer it. Sometimes I told the truth and said our family had four kids, but the usual follow-up question — "What grades are they in?" — always tripped me up. My youngest brother wasn't in school, or at least not in a school like the ones we went to. He lived in something called a hospital school, an hour's drive away. It didn't actually have grades, and he wasn't actually sick; he was there because he was born with something wrong with his brain. Having to explain all this to a kid I'd just met was difficult, so I often said, "I have an older sister and a younger brother." I knew lying was wrong but the lie was easier than the awkward truth. And if the stranger became a friend, I could correct the lie later.

As the years passed, it felt less and less like a lie.

My brother Bill was born with Down syndrome. My parents took him to the Ontario Hospital School at Smiths Falls when he was two and a half, and left him there for the rest of his life. We visited him faithfully as a family every month when we were children. After we grew up, Mom continued the visits, mostly on her own or with Dad. But in our house Bill was an absence, not a presence. He had no clothes in the closet, no toys in the toy chest, no books on the bookshelves. Framed portrait photos of the rest of us as babies hung on the wall of our parents' bedroom. There were none of him — just a snapshot, in profile, framed on Mom's bureau. Our art projects and sports gear and noisy friends filled the house. We saw nothing of his. Yes, he was my brother, but his day-to-day life was utterly separate from mine.

The rupture in my family always troubled me, especially after I had children of my own. As a parent, the idea of sending my toddler to an institution was horrifying. Unimaginable, in fact. Yet my parents, who were kind and loving people, somehow found it justifiable, even reasonable, to exile their youngest child because he had Down syndrome. And they were not alone; thousands of other parents of children with intellectual disabilities had made the same decision. The phrase my parents used to explain it — "Sending Bill to Smiths Falls was the best thing we could have done for him" — became a family mantra of sorts, intoned whenever talk turned to Bill. I heard it countless times growing up, and I sometimes said it myself. No one wanted to believe my parents' well-intentioned decision might have been the wrong one, or that there were other, better, ways for Bill to live. When my own children began to echo it back to me, however, it stopped me cold. By the time they met their uncle Bill, around 1990, the idea of shutting a child away simply because he had Down syndrome sounded like something from the Dark Ages. It was the stuff of nightmares.

I made my living with words, first as a journalist and later as a journalism professor and scholar, and I thought often about writing about Bill over the years. But I rarely talked about it, in large part because I didn't know what I would say. When I retired four or five years ago, many friends and colleagues asked me what I going to *do* with my time. My stock answer was that, after working for forty years, my plan was "to be," not "to do." That was good for a laugh, and it deflected the question nicely. Over coffee one day with a colleague from another university, though, I surprised myself by blurting out a different answer. I told him I was thinking about writing a book about my youngest brother, who grew up in an institution for people with intellectual disabilities and died of a disease he'd caught there. Bill's short life cast a long shadow over my family, before and after my parents sent him away, and I wondered whether it might be time, at long last, to shine some light into that shadow. My colleague responded to the idea enthusiastically.

Over the following months, I began to sound out people I trusted to help me focus my thoughts. One of these discussions took place under the stars and over a bottle (or three) of wine with my good friends Mary Somers and Norma Greenaway, two former journalists with great news judgment and a deep appreciation of the ways of the world. They immediately grasped that Bill's story was more than a story about family, love, and loss; it was part of a larger narrative about disability and social policy. I couldn't tell one story without telling the other.

This meant I needed to understand how the Ontario Hospital School in Smiths Falls — later known as the Rideau Regional Centre — and others like it in Canada, the United States, the United Kingdom, and elsewhere became the standard approach for caring for children with disabilities, why they prevailed for more than a century, and how we finally got rid of them. I also hoped to find out more about Bill. I knew this would be difficult: he had been dead for close to twenty years, and the institution where he lived had shut its doors forever in 2009, long before I launched into this project. But I hoped that telling his story would remind people of how badly all of us — families, bureaucrats, politicians, educators, doctors — responded to the birth of people like Bill. We gave little thought to the possibility that they might enrich our lives, rather than drain our emotional resources. We dehumanized them. We convinced ourselves that banishing them from their families and communities would do them (and us) a kindness, and we turned our backs on the abuse or neglect they suffered in places like Rideau Regional. Our attempt to "solve" the "problem" of intellectual disability by shutting people away in institutions was no solution at all. On the contrary, it led to intolerable injustice.

In 2014, as Bill's closest living relative, I applied to the Ontario ministry in charge of the institutions for whatever information they had about my brother. A heavy package thumped into my mailbox several weeks later with a cover note saying it contained an exact copy of

Bill's resident file. It's twelve hundred pages long, covering pretty well every aspect of his life on the inside. And, frankly, it's kind of a mess. There are no records at all for some years and multiple copies of records for other years. Pages appear out of sequence, and some seem to have been shoved carelessly into the file. A quick example: page 119 is a 1959 "conference report" on Bill's psychometric examination, updated with a single line each in 1969, 1979, and 1982; page 120 is a 1995 permission form to transfer Bill's body to the morgue. Some classes of record start and end for no apparent reason. Some records are contradictory. Many are repetitive, as if copied from a template with just a change in the date. Nonetheless, the records from doctors, infirmary nurses, ward staff, occupational therapists, residential counsellors, work supervisors, medical technicians, and others reveal a lot about Bill's life. They also reveal a lot about how the institutions operated and how they viewed the people who lived in them. Especially in the first half of his life at Smiths Falls, when Ontario's Department of Health was in charge of the institution, the driving principle seems to have been that if you can count it or measure it, put it in his chart; otherwise, don't bother. The individual pieces of the file are peppered with errors — spelling mistakes, mistakes in his name, mistakes on his age (in one report from a doctor, his age is off by twenty years), even medical orders entered in error and struck through later. One of the very first records in the file, from the physician who examined him when he moved into the facility, has an error. It lists the time of Bill's admission as 1:35 a.m., not 1:35 p.m. A small error, but it sets a disturbing tone.

I was able to get Bill's personal file thanks to a recent class-action lawsuit on behalf of former institution residents. The province agreed, as part of the settlement, to create an electronic archive of more than sixty-five thousand scanned documents relating to the operations of the institutions. One set of documents is on a Ministry of Children, Community, and Social Services website, and is heavily redacted to remove any identifying information.[1] Even newspaper clippings, the most public of documents, are blanked out. The unredacted set is available in the Archives of Ontario at York University. Researchers who want to look through it must file a form requesting access to personal information; sign a five-page research agreement promising to keep any personal information in the documents confidential and to refrain from contacting anyone identified in a record without the express permission of the Archives of Ontario; and go to Toronto to work on a dedicated computer in a glass-walled but private room. Researchers cannot print, download, or reproduce documents, though they can take notes. The instructions for using both sets of documents—those on the website and in the archives—say it's possible to search the records by institution, date, or keyword. Keyword searches are limited to the title of the document, however, and many of the document titles are generic. There are hundreds of records titled Medication Incident Form, for example. An injury to a resident may show up as a Resident Incident, Accident and Injury Report, as a Ministry of Community and Social Services—Resident Accident and Injury Report, or as a Contentious Issue Report. The only way to find a particular incident is to go through them one by one. A search of Rideau Regional records also calls up similar documents from the Huronia and the Southwestern Ontario regional centres. Some records appear a half-dozen times. Many of the records are cover letters that have been separated from other documents, and it is virtually impossible to put the cover letter and the document together. It takes high-level research skills, enormous patience, and hours of work to get much out of the database. These documents, along with Bill's personal file, form the basis of this book.

I also spoke with a number of people—former staff members, families of former residents, key figures in the class-action suits, scholars, experts in community living, and my own family—who either knew Bill or had their own experiences with the institutions. Some shared only happy memories, though they were in the minority. Some of the former staff had been witnesses to abuse. Others, as part of their jobs, had to treat the people they worked with in ways that made them uncomfortable. Some sources corroborated my own memories, confirmed or corrected my impressions, or filled in gaps in my knowledge. Others added to what I already knew about Bill's life. This book deals with sensitive material, and I was concerned about invading the privacy or former staff members, residents, or their families, as well as about digging up sad memories. I decided to give sources approval over any quotations of theirs that I used. I also decided not to publish the identity of anyone named in Bill's residential file.

Back when I began thinking seriously about how to write about Bill, I mentioned the idea to some other friends and colleagues and got some surprising reactions. One friend asked whether I was angry with my parents and trying to get back at them. Another wanted to know whether I was feeling guilty about Bill. No, I replied to the first. Of course not, I replied to the second.

The anger came later. So did the guilt, and the regret. I wish I had been able to talk to my parents about how they felt when other families won the battle to keep their children at home and send them to the public schools, or why they rejected the idea of moving Bill out of the institution when they had the chance, or whether they had any regrets about splitting up their family. I don't believe, however, that I could have written this story while my parents were alive. My mother struggled until the day she died with guilt and despair over abandoning her baby. My father swallowed his feelings about Bill and rarely spoke of him. Getting them to confront the full implications of the choices they made for their son would have been cruel. Some stories, they believed, are too personal to share. But that makes them all the more compelling to tell.

Chapter 1

"THE GREAT **MONGOLIAN** FAMILY"

My parents met in the operating room at the Ottawa Civic Hospital in 1943. She was a registered nurse, and he was a very young intern. It was not a case of love at first sight. "She whacked me over the fingers with a Kelly forcep because I was messing up her instrument tray," my father recalled of their first encounter.[1] But their eyes met over their surgical masks, and romance soon followed.

My mother, Dorothy King, grew up in North Bay, Ontario, in a family that came to Canada with few prospects and less education. Her grandparents, John and Alice Annie King, emigrated from England in the 1880s as indentured farm workers. John signed his marriage certificate with an X, so we know they were illiterate.[2] After a year or two working on a farm near Ottawa to pay off their passage across the Atlantic, the family wandered north, where John found work as a track inspector for the Canadian Pacific Railway. He died just a few years later, leaving Alice with five young children, including a lean, dark eleven-year-old named Albert, who would grow up to be Dorothy's father and my grandfather. I don't know how far Albert got in school; his youngest brother, Ernie, made it to grade six. As soon as they were old enough, the King boys got jobs. Albert became a railway switchman and a yardman. Eventually, he earned enough to marry his sweetheart, Mary McLaren, a farmer's daughter from a remote region of Parry Sound, who had moved to North Bay as a teenager to work as a cook.

Albert and Mary had two boys, followed by two girls. The youngest girl died in infancy, which meant that Dorothy, born in 1920, was the baby of the family and the only daughter. Dorothy was smart, beautiful, and a bit brash. She had raven hair, arched black brows over sea-green eyes, and an imperious tilt to her chin. Like most working-class girls of her era, she learned how to sew, and started making her own clothes when she was in her teens. She had a good eye for design and was skilled with a needle and thread, and she managed to turn scraps into something beautiful. The Kings were poor, but so was everyone else they knew once the Great Depression set in. And her family was better off than many — at least her father had a job.

In June of 1934, Dorothy's safe world fell apart. On a weekend fishing trip to Bull Frog Lake near Mattawa, her father fell ill. Within hours, he was dead. Dorothy told me she believed the cause was a perforated ulcer. A newspaper clipping from the time said it was a burst appendix, while the coroner's report said the cause of death was an acute intestinal blockage, though no autopsy was held.[3] Whatever the cause, Albert King was gone at the age of forty-eight.

Like the Kings of the previous generation, Albert's family found ways to scrape by. His widow, Mary, took in other family members to help with expenses on their house. Dorothy, who turned fourteen a few weeks before her father died, stayed in school and longed for a bigger life. She dreamed of a world where women wore gowns and jewels and rode in fine cars through cities that lit up at night, where poor girls with good looks, smart tongues, and hearts of gold married millionaires. She fed these dreams with the movies that came through town, and wrote fan letters to Hollywood stars. Jean Harlow sent her a signed photo, which Dorothy kept until she died.

She knew, however, that her choices were limited. Wife, teacher, secretary, or nurse — those were the only paths open to girls like Dorothy. Of the four, nurse sounded most promising. She would have to leave home to go to nursing school, and that was fine with her. Nurses wore crisp uniforms, which meant her homemade wardrobe wouldn't matter. They worked in hospitals that were clean and white, nothing like the grimy rail yards where she grew up. Self-possessed, fastidious, and cool-headed in a crisis, Dorothy thought she'd like the work and would be good at it, too. And she thought doctors would make better husbands than railroad men. As soon as she could manage it, she packed her bags and headed south to the nursing school at the Ottawa Civic Hospital.

Doug McKercher, my father, grew up in the general store in tiny Vernon, Ontario, about twenty miles south of Ottawa. His mother, Bessie, was the youngest of ten children; Sandy Stewart, their father, was a prosperous local farmer, Baptist deacon, justice of the peace, and proud sheep breeder. Doug's father, Bert, came from the large Scottish community in nearby Glengarry County, and moved to Vernon when he was still a teenager to manage a local bank branch. Bert and Bessie married in March 1918, a few months before Bert was drafted.[4] He spent the final days of the First World War in London, as a clerk in the War Office. By all accounts he loved it, but he came home to Bessie in 1919 and settled into life as a merchant. Doug was born in 1921; his brother John two years later.

Bert's business included a general store, bank, post office, and filling station, and it did well despite the onset of the Depression. His family life was much less successful. Bert was a dreamer, yearning for a more glamorous life than weighing potatoes and trying to keep the bugs out of the raisin bin. He was also a drinker—a cardinal sin in Bessie's family of teetotallers. Worst of all, he had a roving eye.

Trapped in an unhappy marriage with two growing sons, Bessie often turned to her sister Annie for advice. Annie had a rich husband and no children of her own. Knowing Annie, I am sure she drove Bert crazy, but she was always there for Bessie and her boys, sometimes in unexpected ways. She taught Doug golf because she thought gentlemen should play golf, or at least know how to behave on the golf course. She advised Bessie on how to handle her household. She bailed out Bessie financially when

Bert walked out for good in late 1938 or early 1939, rejoining the army and leaving a pile of debt. Most significantly for my family, she paid Doug's tuition to Queen's University.

Annie thought Doug should be a doctor. Bessie agreed, and so did Doug. In fact, he said many times he never thought of doing anything else. In the fall of 1938, Annie drove him to Kingston to join the Queen's University School of Medicine's class of '44. He was one of the youngest in his class, but he managed the pressures of medical school with relative ease. Compared to Vernon, Kingston was positively cosmopolitan. Queen's was full of smart, young people who worked hard but made time for dances, parties, and hockey games too. Doug, who was athletic and always up for a party, loved it. Many of the young doctors he studied with became life-long friends. When the Second World War broke out, Queen's accelerated its medical training, keeping students in school year-round so they could move into military service as quickly as possible. This meant Doug finished medical school a year early, in 1943, at the age of twenty-one. He had signed up with the Royal Canadian Navy—Dorothy often joked that he chose the navy because he liked the uniforms—and his active service would begin right after a short internship. Bessie was living in Ottawa by this time, working for the federal government, and Doug decided to intern at the Ottawa Civic Hospital.

And so Doug—and his soon-to-be-rapped knuckles—met Dorothy.

Within months they were engaged, and within the year Doug was gone to sea. He was surgeon-lieutenant on the HMCS *Strathadam*, a frigate plowing back and forth across the Atlantic. He rarely talked to his children about his wartime experiences, though we know they stayed with him. After he died, I found his discharge papers from the navy in his wallet. He had kept them for more than sixty years.

When Doug was eighty-nine, Ottawa newspaper columnist Dave Brown interviewed him about his war. Brown's story begins with one of Doug's favourite wartime tales about how he, a very young doctor stationed in Halifax, and an even younger RCMP officer tracked down a prostitute with distinctive tattoos and a virulent case of venereal disease.

Doug called it "the great butterfly hunt" after one of her tattoos. He smiled as he told the story, adding with a twinkle that this was how he won the war. Brown commented, "Most that experienced war are that way. They keep a light story near the top of the memory in case anybody asks. It takes a little patience for the scars to show." Doug gave him a peek at some of those scars, recalling the horror when his ship sank a German submarine in the Irish Sea. "What an awful way to die," he said. "And so unnecessary. The era of the wolf packs was long gone and that sub was just loitering around. The war was almost over. They weren't much of a threat. Sometimes in the middle of the night, I think of them down there. Entombed." While attacking another sub some months later, the depth charges on the deck of the *Strathadam* exploded prematurely. Six men died, a dozen more were wounded, and the shock waves stunned the officers on the open bridge, Doug included. As ship's doctor, Doug took care of the wounded. But the deaths haunted him. "We marched behind our dead to a cemetery in Londonderry. We gave them a military funeral, and then in formation, marched out. As I turned my back, I could hear the dirt hitting the coffins. Funny. That sound still comes back in the middle of the night."[5]

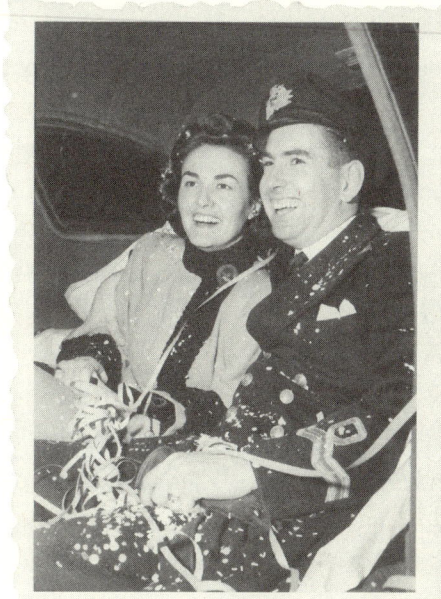

A quick, wartime wedding in Halifax led to a marriage that lasted for 50 years. Despite disagreeing over what to do about their youngest son, Doug and Dorothy remained in love until the end.

The accident left Doug with some permanent hearing loss. But as the war in Europe drew to an end, he felt lucky to have survived, ready to start a new life, and eager to share it with Dorothy.

During one of his rare leaves in the fall of 1945, Dorothy flew to Halifax and they married. It was a quick, wartime ceremony: he wore dress blues, she a wine-red suit with velvet trim. Aside from Doug, Dorothy knew nobody at her wedding. The best man was a stranger, and the maid of honour was an acquaintance of Doug's who wore her nursing uniform to the ceremony. No family members attended. Doug's father, Bert, was long gone from his son's life, and his mother was working full-time in Ottawa. Dorothy's father was dead, and her mother was too ill to travel; she would die of cancer the following year, at the age of fifty-three. How strange it was, Dorothy told my sister Mary years later, to feel so lonely and so happy at the same time. Their honeymoon was a few days at the Cornwallis Inn in Kentville, Nova Scotia. Then Doug had to get back to work.

Doug wanted to become a specialist: an ear, nose, and throat doctor. After his discharge from the navy, Dorothy followed him through four years of residencies and specialization courses in Halifax, Montreal, London (Ontario), and St. Louis, Missouri. The doctor he studied with in St. Louis wanted them to settle there, but Dorothy said no. They set their sights on Ottawa, where Bessie lived and they felt welcome in the medical community. In 1949, his specialist training completed, Doug signed on as junior partner to a gentlemanly Scottish-born doctor, J.K. Milne Dickie, who was one of the city's best—and best-known—specialists. Dorothy almost immediately got pregnant. Bessie, now and ever after known as Nana, was thrilled.

Though my parents started their family late, by the spring of 1956 they had made up for lost time. The family now included fair-haired and blue-eyed Mary, a serious six-year-old with a well-developed sense of right and wrong; four-year-old me, dark-haired and brown-eyed, with bad tonsils but a good attitude toward life; and Bob, a handsome and sensitive two-year-old with dark hair and Dad's hazel-brown eyes. Dorothy was pregnant again, and she and Doug were hoping for another son. They pictured the two boys sharing the big, double-sized bedroom at the end of the hall in the house they were building, in a new suburb in Ottawa's west end — the first and only house they would own.

Mom was good at being pregnant. She once told me it made her feel healthy and alive, and she loved watching her belly grow and dreaming about the baby. But this pregnancy was difficult. Dad's job was to build his practice and bring home an income; hers was to take care of everything else. She was raising three children under six, one still in diapers, and she was in charge of equipping and furnishing our new house. I was too young to have any idea of the pressures she faced, but I am certain she felt overwhelmed. Mom was the kind of person who fretted over details the rest of us wouldn't even notice. She wanted her house, her wardrobe, her children, and her life to be, in one of her favourite phrases, "well groomed." Any deviation from that standard was a failure.

As her due date approached, she said later, she felt apprehensive. She lost weight during the last month of pregnancy rather than gaining it, and that worried her. She went into labour on September 6, and the delivery was pretty quick. Like Mary and me, this baby came into the world fanny first. He weighed six pounds, three ounces — quite a bit less than the rest of us, who were all eight-pounders or more. As soon as she woke from the pre-delivery anesthetic — routine practice in those days — Mom knew something was wrong. She spotted a flag on her chart; as a nurse, she knew it signified a problem. No one came over to her bed to congratulate her. Instead, the nurses avoided making eye contact. She lay there alone, woozy and afraid until, finally, her obstetrician came over to her.

I'm sorry, Dorothy, he said. *It's a boy, but he's a mongoloid.*

—

No one uses the term *mongoloid* today except as an insult. But in the
1950s, it was widely accepted, even by the World Health Organization and
advocacy groups for people with intellectual impairments. In fact, John
Langdon Down himself applied it to the disability that now carries his
name.[6] Down, then the superintendent of the Royal Earlswood Asylum
for Idiots, published an article in 1866 connecting selected disabilities
with the branches of humanity identified by the German anthropologist
J.F. Blumenbach: Caucasians, Mongolians, Aztecs, Malayans, and
Ethiopians. Down tried to assign Earlswood residents to one or another
category. "Of course, there are numerous representatives of the great
Caucasian family," he wrote. He also identified several of the "Ethiopian
variety," characterized by thick lips and woolly hair. In those of English
or European descent, he wrote, the "Ethiopian variety" showed up as
"specimens of white negroes." He identified Malay and indigenous
North American varieties, the former with soft, black, curly hair and
large mouths and the latter with prominent cheeks, deep-set eyes, and a
"slightly apish nose." But the group that interested him most belonged
to "the great Mongolian family," in large part due to the size of that
particular group. "The Mongolian type of idiocy occurs in more than ten
per cent of the cases which are presented to me," he wrote.

Down's taxonomy was more than an exercise in Victorian racism,
though racist it certainly was. Down was an abolitionist. "If these great
racial divisions are fixed and definite," he mused in the final paragraph
of his essay, "how comes it that disease is able to break down the barrier,
and to simulate so closely the features of the members of another
division."[7] In other words, if white parents could have children who were
"Mongolian"—or "Ethiopian" or "Malay," for that matter—then white
people had no natural right to enslave people with brown or black skin.
Down's racial taxonomy never caught on and he eventually abandoned
it, but it made an important contribution in another way: it recognized
that people with this disability he called Mongolian are born that way,
and that the disability follows a pattern.

Almost a century later, scientists would discover the genetic basis of the patterns Down observed. The vast majority of people with Down syndrome — something like 95 per cent of them[8] — have forty-seven chromosomes in each cell of their body, not forty-six like the rest of us. That forty-seventh is a third, or extra, copy of a specific chromosome, number 21, and it's present from conception or shortly thereafter. Down syndrome is not the only congenital condition with a trisomy, or three copies, of a chromosome: Edwards syndrome, also known as trisomy 18, and Patau syndrome, or trisomy 13, have also been identified, as have trisomies of all or parts of chromosomes 8, 9, and 22. All cause a range of birth defects, including intellectual deficits. Trisomies may also occur in the X and Y sex chromosomes, with varying effects.

Down was correct in noting that the disability is the most common genetically based cause of intellectual impairment in humans, but exactly how common is difficult to pin down. The World Health Organization estimates that Down syndrome shows up in one in 1,000 to 1,100 births worldwide. The US Centers for Disease Control traditionally uses a somewhat higher incidence, one in 700, and reports that the number of American babies born with Down syndrome increased by about 30 per cent between 1979 and 2003. A 2013 report from the Public Health Agency of Canada sets the incidence at about one in 800 births. A 2016 Harvard Medical School statistical analysis estimates that the number of Americans living with Down syndrome quadrupled between 1950 and 2010, going up to 206,366, mainly because of higher life expectancies. The Canadian Down Syndrome Society estimates that 45,000 Canadians are living with the disorder.[9]

Why Down syndrome happens no one knows, though the age of the mother is a factor. According to the US Centers for Disease Control, the odds of having a child with the disorder are almost five times higher in older mothers than in younger ones.[10] The risk creeps up slowly until a woman reaches thirty-five, and then accelerates. By the time a woman is forty, her chances of having a child with Down syndrome are about one in eighty. But, because younger women are more likely to have babies than older ones, the bulk of people with Down syndrome are born to women who are under thirty-five.

Down syndrome affects boys and girls and appears in all classes, ethnic groups, and cultures, on all continents, and throughout history. A seven-thousand-year-old Greek figurine may be the oldest representation of the disorder in Western art.[11] In 2014, scientists argued furiously over whether ancient bones found on the Indonesian island of Flores were those of someone with Down syndrome, rather than bones from a primitive species of hominin. The Down syndrome side lost the argument, but the very fact it took place underlines our understanding that the disorder has probably been around for about as long as we have.[12]

The distinctive genetic structure of Down syndrome shows up in a distinctive set of physical characteristics, and Mom's obstetrician recognized them instantly. The new baby was fair-haired like Mary, and his eyes would be hazel-brown like Bob's, but he looked much more like other children with Down syndrome than he did like the rest of us. Down made the same observation about his patients: "So marked is this, that when placed side by side, it is difficult to believe that the specimens compared are not children of the same parents."[13] The baby's face and nose were flat, and he had deep-set, slanted eyes, with a characteristic fold in the eyelids. His head was small. So was his mouth, though his tongue was thick and stuck out through his lips. His hands were also small, and he had a single crease across the palm, not two creases like the rest of us. (Down's son Reginald is credited with associating that detail — he called it the "simian crease" — with Down syndrome. *Simian* means "ape-like," which tells you a lot about Reginald's view of these people.[14]) The baby had poor muscle tone: his lower lip was slack, his reflexes were slow.

The visual cues were unmistakable, even in a newborn, but there was more. Half the children born with Down syndrome have cardiac abnormalities. My brother was one of them: he had a heart murmur. Weakened immune systems are also common in children with Down syndrome. In the days before antibiotics and advanced surgical techniques, most babies with the syndrome died in infancy or early childhood. Even as late as the 1960s, the average life span of a child with Down syndrome was about ten years. Today it's about sixty years.[15]

The biggest concerns surrounding Billy's future, though, weren't physical. The extra chromosome meant the baby would have an intellectual impairment. It also meant that from the moment of his birth, Down syndrome would define my brother's life. He would never be seen, not even by his parents, as a child who happened to have a disability. In the eyes of his family, the medical establishment, the education system, social service providers, and governments at all levels, he was a defective child. And something would have to be done about him.

—

The pressure to send my brother to the new Ontario Hospital School in Smiths Falls, which had opened in 1951, began almost the moment he arrived. Friends who knew of, or had, a child with an intellectual disability visited Mom while she was still in the hospital recovering from the birth. They urged her to send him to an institution. A psychiatrist who didn't know them, but who was the father of one of their friends, telephoned Dad and told him not to let Mom bring the baby home. It would only make sending Billy away harder, he said. Better to send him to an institution now, so everyone could get on with their lives.

In his history of Down syndrome, McGill University professor David Wright recalls that his parents faced much the same pressure a decade later, when his sister was born in 1967. After confirming that the infant was "a mongoloid"—the term was still in use then, though it had begun to go out of fashion—the obstetrician asked whether the parents wanted to take her home. His mother's deadpan response was, "Isn't that what you do with your children?" The doctor's question, Wright adds, "was far from extraordinary."[16]

For his family, as in mine, the argument in favour of institutionalization had its own perverse and complex logic. It went something like this: it would be best for the child to be raised with others of his own kind, where he would grow up as one among equals rather than as the child who would forever lag behind his siblings. In the institution, he would get the specialized care and training that would allow him to develop to his full, albeit limited, potential. Keeping him at home would deny him of that specialized care and training. Instead, he could only watch, with growing resentment, as his siblings achieved things he never could. If it would be hard on the "retarded child," it would be no picnic for the other children in the family either. According to Wright, "It was commonly assumed amongst self-styled educational experts that the presence of a severely disabled child would divert emotional energy from the other children, leading to psycho-social and developmental problems in siblings of Down's Syndrome children."[17] The inevitable outcome would be jealousy, conflict, and heartbreak, and the sooner the family got rid of the child who was causing the problem, the better off everyone would be.

Remarkably little actual research substantiated this view. One of the leading scholars of the post-war years, Ann Gath, cited early studies that showed having a child with an intellectual disability at home was a burden for families, especially for mothers.[18] A 1957 study found that 15 per cent of siblings were adversely affected. A 1962 American study suggested that parents played a critical role in how well other children adapted. If the parents agreed on how to handle the child with an intellectual disability, the other children went along with whatever they decided. If the parents disagreed, the siblings were more likely to show disturbances. Gath's own research found that siblings of a child with Down syndrome were twice as likely to become anti-social, have difficulty making friends, act miserably or disobediently, or have temper tantrums. Sisters were more affected than brothers, and older sisters more than younger ones. None of these studies was particularly decisive or convincing, but they fed into prevailing social attitudes of the era.

By the time Wright's sister was born, the "send-them-to-an-institution" argument was starting to lose traction. But in 1956, the year my brother was born, the thought of raising a child with intellectual disabilities at home with his brothers and sisters amounted to heresy among the people in my parents' world, a throwback to an uncivilized age. Instead, my parents were told they should be grateful that the newest, largest, and most up-to-date "hospital school" in Ontario was just a short drive away, in Smiths Falls. This meant they could solve the problem my new brother posed and, if they wished, still stay in touch with him. They probably did not know that the new hospital school was already overcrowded, and that the wait list for spots at Smiths Falls and at the older institution in Orillia had seventeen hundred names on it that fall.[19]

Devastated and overwhelmed, Mom didn't know what to do. She was also feeling the first stirrings of a crushing guilt she would bear for the rest of her life. Her head filled with questions. Was it all her fault? Had she jinxed things by being ungrateful to be pregnant this time? Had she waited too long to start her family? Should she have stopped at three children? What had she done wrong? Dad had no answers, and no clear idea about what to do next. But as a doctor, he took the advice of his fellow doctors and other experts seriously. And the experts all said the same thing: he and Dorothy should send the child away, and they should do so sooner rather than later.

Days after Mom came home and while the baby was still in the hospital, Dad phoned Dr. Harold Frank, the superintendent of the Ontario Hospital School at Smiths Falls. He had one question: Would the institution admit a newborn? If the answer was yes, the new baby might well have disappeared from the family before he ever joined it. The answer was no. "So that was one decision made for us," Mom said.

They brought the baby home.

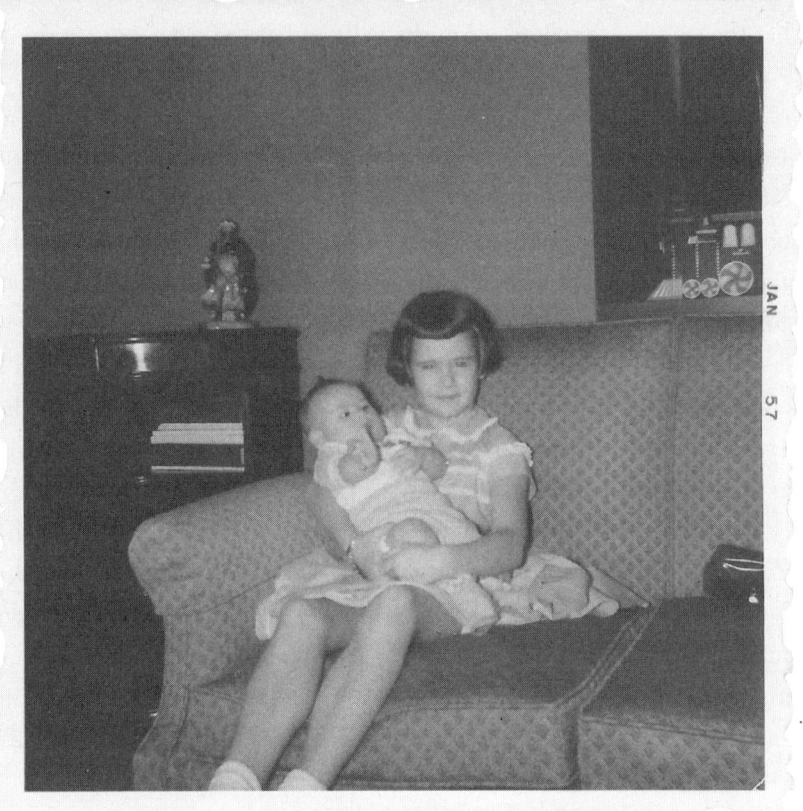

Bill had to stay in the hospital for a while after his birth,
but he was home and settled in well before Christmas — and
content to pose for photos in my sister Mary's arms.

Chapter 2

"A DARLING, **EASY BABY**"

My parents knew hundreds of people around Ottawa and had scores of friends, but they knew only one family that had kept their intellectually impaired child at home. Mom and Dad had no idea how Mary, Bob, and I would react to the baby, or how our friends might, or how their own friends would react, though they feared a good number of those reactions would be negative. None of the fast-growing families in our booming neighbourhood had a child like this, and Mom and Dad had little idea, beyond the common-sense experience of being parents to three kids already, of how to raise a fragile baby with Down syndrome.

Even coming up with a name for the newborn was difficult. My sister was named for our grandmothers, Mary and Elizabeth. Dad named me after a favourite patient, a little girl called Cathy Ann. Luckily, Aunt Annie and Kathleen Dickie, the sister of Dad's medical partner and my self-appointed godmother, could stake some claim to the name as well. My brother, Robert Douglas, got Dad's name and the name of a Scottish king. For this baby, Mom once told me, the priority was finding a name that wouldn't offend anyone. No one, she said, wants to have a child with Down syndrome named after them.

They settled on William Andrew. Dad had a few Williams in his family, including an uncle who drowned at the age of eighteen and a first cousin who wasn't close enough to feel my parents had named the baby after him. William was a popular choice — it was number six on the list of top baby boy names in the 1950s[1] — and Andrew was the patron saint of Scotland. We never called my brother William. He was Billy when he was a baby, Bill when he got older, and Boo when we were goofing around.

Billy had to stay in the hospital for a while after Mom went home — I am not sure why or for how long — but, once they brought him home, he settled into our house quickly. "He was a darling, easy baby — never cried — and despite being slow to smile and later on sit up, each advance was a triumph," Mom later recalled. "There was no question of him leaving us because he was a loved part of the family. Life went on with no problems."[2] I am sure she was sincere when she wrote those words in a letter to Mary, Bob, and me, but in just about every way possible, Billy was treated differently, even within the family. The rest of us were treated differently, as a family, because of Bill. And the question of him leaving us was very much on the table.

When the rest of us were born, our parents announced our arrivals in the *Ottawa Journal* as soon after the birth as possible. Bob's birth announcement, for example, appeared in the July 6 edition, less than forty-eight hours after his birth: "To Dr. and Mrs. D.D. McKercher at the Ottawa Civic Hospital on Sunday July 4, 1954, a son." A modest announcement, yes, but full of pride. With Bill, there was no announcement. I scanned two months of newspapers and found nothing. The flood of cards and flowers and baby gifts that greeted the arrival of the other McKercher children didn't materialize. People didn't know what to say about this baby, so most said nothing. Close friends of my parents greeted the birth with expressions of sympathy, not celebration. Acquaintances averted their eyes. Strangers stared or asked personal questions — not necessarily rude questions, but intrusive ones nonetheless. The kids in the neighbourhood were curious to see Billy. Their parents had probably warned them that he was "different," and not in a good way. The other kids rarely said cruel things to our faces, but I am sure they snickered behind our backs about the strange new baby in our house.

What we were experiencing was anything but uncommon for families like ours. The stigma of what was called "mental retardation" in those post-war years ran deep, like the stigmas associated then with alcoholism or cancer. All three conditions were cause for personal shame, so much so that people rarely spoke the words aloud in polite company; they whispered. Having a child with an intellectual disability was at best an embarrassment and at worst a sign of something rotten behind the facade of a happy family. "Historically, it has carried a mark of shame, identifying the afflicted as a subhuman creature, a vegetable, or a blob of flesh," according to Peter Tyor and Leland Bell, authors of a leading history of intellectual disability in the United States. "Tortured and dismayed by this reality, parents and relatives of the retarded have been overwhelmed with feelings of guilt, failure and futility, and they, too, suffer social stigmatization."[3] In conservative, Protestant Ontario, the stigma had religious overtones based on the Old Testament idea that sin could be passed on from one generation to another. It would be hard to imagine greater evidence of parental sin than a son with an intellectual disability. The traditional solution, as Tyor and Bell describe, was to send someone like Billy to an institution where, "out of sight and shunned as an outcast, the child—and later adult—can be forgotten."[4] My parents would not have put the institutional option in quite these terms. They would have emphasized the positive: the institution could take on the burden of giving their disabled son the care he'd need for what they expected would be a short life. That he *was* a burden, however, was taken for granted; they never saw him as anything else. Darling and easy though he might have been, tiny Billy was a family tragedy.

—

When we were very young, before Bill was born and before we moved to the new house in the suburbs, Mom and Dad took us to Parkdale United Church every Sunday. In nice weather, we walked the few blocks to get there. If it was cold or wet, we took the car. We were not a particularly religious family, but our parents believed going to church was good for everyone. Parkdale United is part of a liberal Protestant denomination that sees infant baptism as a first step toward joining the community of the church. Baptism day was part consecration and part celebration, a fancy-dress occasion for the entire family, and in my family it typically happened when the child was about six months old. This means that Billy, born in the fall of 1956, should have been baptized in the spring of 1957. He was not. I have no idea why our parents decided against baptism that spring. Granted, his health was delicate and his life expectancy unknown, but I suspect that another, darker reason accounted for their decision to hold off. Baptizing Billy would have meant standing up at the front of the church and publicly claiming him as their child, as an equal to their other children, and as someone who would eventually have a unique and personal place in the church and in the broader community. I don't think Dad or Mom ever saw him that way.

In fact, over years of conversations with both my parents, I was often struck by how they talked about Bill's relationship to the world beyond home. They rarely took him to new places, either as a child or an adult. The reason they usually gave was that they didn't want to make "other people" feel uncomfortable. Once or twice, I pressed the issue. Why should anyone care what strangers think, I'd say, and why would strangers feel uncomfortable around Bill anyway? The answer, almost invariably, was that these "other people" might be nervous or ill at ease or uncertain about how to talk to Bill. This went double for "other children," who might, my parents said, find him frightening.

The idea that my brother was somehow monstrous permeated much of what my parents said about him, not just in the 1950s but throughout his life. When Bill was an adult, Mom took him to Burger King at off-peak hours to limit the number of other diners he would encounter. "One day some older ladies had stopped for lunch and as we left he whacked each of them on the shoulder to say goodbye," she recalled. "Talk about looks of terror!"[5] I doubt they were really terrified, though I am certain my mother was embarrassed. After I moved back to Ottawa in the late 1980s, I regularly suggested that I go with Mom the next time she visited Bill. Mom almost always found a reason why this wasn't a good idea. The excuses sounded logical on the surface, but they concealed a deep fear that unpredictable Bill would somehow disgust me or embarrass her. I told her my husband, Vinny, would like to meet him, too, and so would our daughters. Again and again, she demurred. But eventually, reluctantly, cautiously, she relented. I reconnected with him first, then Vinny met him. When I finally convinced her that our girls should meet their Uncle Bill, Mom fretted for weeks before saying yes. She worried about how to prepare them beforehand, and offered suggestions about how to debrief them afterward — actually using the word *debrief,* which made me laugh. (She didn't think it was funny.) She was especially anxious that Bill might scare the girls, or give them nightmares. None of that happened. We all went to the Hershey factory that day, and Bill and the kids bonded over chocolate. Rosemary and Madeline were glad to meet this mysterious uncle they had heard about all their lives, curious about his disability, and interested in learning about him. Bill was happy to meet them, too. This first visit went well enough that a few others followed, and Mom and Dad even brought the girls to a family day at the institution one year when Vinny and I were away. Rosemary particularly appreciated the chance to spend time with him, saying her visits with Bill gave her a deeper sense of empathy for lives unlike her own.

My parents believed in good manners and proper behaviour in public. But Mom and Dad's concern for "other people" was, to a significant degree, a ruse — a way of deflecting their own shame and embarrassment about Bill. Dad, especially, did not see Bill as someone to be celebrated or shown off to friends and acquaintances. Fed and clothed properly, of course. Cared for, certainly. Hugged and kissed like the rest of us when he came home from work, naturally. But passed proudly from arm to arm at a post-christening party in the church reception hall? Impossible.

—

Every Sunday afternoon in the summer, we drove to Nana's cottage on the Rideau River, about twenty miles south of our house. We always stopped on the way at a country store for ice cream and worms—dished out by the same clerk, which made Mom shudder. At Nana's we played croquet on the back lawn, took turns in the rowboat, and fished off the dock, hooking and tossing back dozens of small perch, sunfish, and bass. Great-aunt Ella, a retired nurse who never married and lived with Nana, was always there. Ella actually owned the cottage, but to us it was always Nana's. Uncle John's growing family often came, too. Almost every year in the early 1950s, one of the McKercher brothers had a new baby who spent summer Sunday afternoons lying on a blanket in the shade of the big willow tree. Neighbours or friends who dropped by would have a chance to meet—and admire—the latest addition to Nana's brood.

But not Billy. When someone dropped by, Ella scooped him up and hustled him inside the cottage. This infuriated Mom, but as Ella saw it, having Billy outside with the rest of us when company dropped by was unseemly, socially offensive, and an invitation to mean-spirited gossip. Hiding him inside would be better for all of us.

To Mary, Bob, and me, though, Billy was just another baby. Mary and I knew there was something not right about him. Six- and four-year-olds are pretty good at picking up on the tone of adult conversations—*Such a shame... What a tragedy... Too bad... He's sweet now while he's little, but what will he be like later?... What are you going to* do *with him?*—if not on the precise meaning of what they overhear. We all learned the word *mongoloid*: even Bob, who, at two, was just starting to speak. Mom explained that it was the correct term for someone like Billy, and much more polite than any of the other cruel words we were likely to hear people use to describe him. I can remember instructing my friends on the proper pronunciation even though we had very little idea of what the word meant, exactly. And life inside the family went along pretty smoothly.

Until the spring of 1958, when it didn't any more.

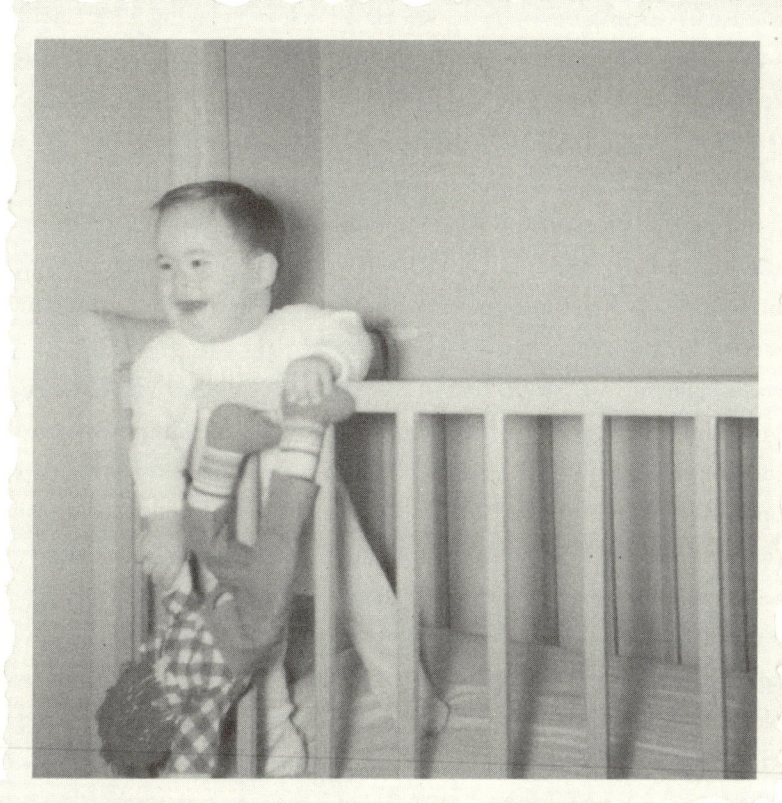

My favourite photo — and favourite memory — of Bill, laughing in the crib
after his nap. He awoke full of fun and ready to take on the world.

At eighteen months, Billy was a small but husky toddler with shiny,
light brown hair and a smile that lit up the room. He had survived a
serious bout of pneumonia at sixteen months — treated at home as his
temperature soared to a frightening 105 degrees — and had just recovered
from the chicken pox, which we all had that year. He was walking,
though in a peculiar way that I can only describe as a tippy-toed shuffle.
He couldn't go up or down stairs, but he got around our ranch-style bungalow just fine. He was learning how to feed himself, though he needed
help. He understood a few words and made sounds that held out the

promise of turning into words some day. He loved playing with crayons, and was learning their colours. He also loved being around the older kids. We found him to be a great audience, laughing hysterically and almost on demand when we did something silly. I especially liked going into his room to get him up from his nap. He'd grab onto the bars of his crib, scramble to his feet, and bounce up and down. I'd bounce in front of him too, and we would laugh until we were both out of breath. At that point he'd flop down into the crib, and I'd flop on the floor, which only made us laugh harder.

But that spring, for no reason our parents could identify, he began vomiting. There was nothing violent about it; he simply spat up a tablespoon or two of foul-smelling goo a dozen or more times a day. He vomited in his crib in the morning, before his afternoon nap, after his afternoon nap, and on and off throughout the night. He vomited before meals and after meals. If we got him bouncing, he'd vomit. If he laughed, he'd vomit. But he also vomited when he was sitting still, or when he was walking from one side of the room to the other. He vomited when he was colouring a picture, or playing with a toy, or cuddling on Mom's lap. He left little puddles of vomit on the floor, on the high chair, on the seats of chairs, on the couch, in the car, on Mom.

The vomit stank. His crib stank. He stank.

When their pediatrician ran out of ideas about what was going on, Mom and Dad admitted Billy to the hospital for tests. What was happening with Billy was not unheard of; babies with Down syndrome often have gastro-intestinal issues. The US National Down Syndrome Society reports that about 5 per cent of children with the condition are born with an intestinal obstruction, which has to be corrected surgically. A smaller number, about 1 per cent, have a fistula that causes their windpipe and their esophagus to be improperly connected. Again, surgery can fix those. Up to 15 per cent have Hirschsprung's disease, where a lack of certain nerve cells in their large intestine leads to severe and chronic constipation and bowel obstruction, and about 3 per cent are born without an anus. And some, between 1 and 5 per cent, have something called gastroesophageal reflux disease, or GERD, in which the muscular ring at the bottom of the esophagus, the clamp that holds food inside the stomach, fails to stay clamped. This failure, which may be related to poor muscle tone, allows the stomach's contents to wash back up the esophagus, and out.[6] Quite possibly, GERD was Billy's problem. In 1958, though, the explanation for his vomiting was that he had a short esophagus. The doctors said they could do nothing about it, and Billy would, they predicted, outgrow it—eventually.

Life got much more complicated after that.

Before, Billy had had the run of the house, like the rest of us. The sunny living room with the grass-green carpet and pale green couch was grown-up territory. On winter afternoons, when the sun streamed in the big west-facing windows, I liked to lie on the rug and pretend I was lying on summer grass. None of us spent much time there otherwise, but now Billy was banned from it. His world contracted to the kitchen, his high chair in the dining room, his crib, and the family room we called the den. The den was where we did most of our living. We kept our toys and games in the cabinet under the TV, and Mom and Dad would have after-dinner coffee and cigarettes in the den while we played and argued over which TV show to watch. The den had an easy-to-clean cork floor—an asset once Bill started vomiting. Mom carried tissues in her pocket at all times, and we all learned to walk around the house with eyes on the floor for fear of slipping in one of Bill's puddles. We always checked the chairs before sitting down. Mom changed the sheets in his crib several times a day, and dressed and redressed him constantly. But sooner or later—usually sooner—almost everything he touched was sticky and smelled of vomit.

"During this time we couldn't take Bill anywhere, even to Nana's, because of the spitting up," Mom recalled. "I remember taking him to the barber one day and he was so cute, sitting up in the chair and smiling at everyone. Suddenly he spit up on the barber's apron and a look of disgust came on everyone's face. After that the barber came to our house."[7] Surely no one would be all that disgusted by a bit of spit-up from a toddler; other customers would probably have ignored it, especially if they had kids of their own. Even so, an apology and a generous tip would have settled things. It seems the one who was most upset by this incident was Mom herself. Fastidious in everything she did and nervous about taking Billy out in public anyway, she must have felt deeply embarrassed, maybe even humiliated, by her son's uncontrollable and messy impulses.

A month passed, and Billy was still vomiting. Three months. Six months. The problem showed no signs of going away.

Taking care of Billy became increasingly time-consuming, adding hours to Mom and Dad's already tight schedule. Mary and I were both in school, she in grade three and me in grade one. Mom had to get us up, dressed, fed, and out the door in time to walk to school, almost a mile away. On particularly frigid mornings, she drove us. Dad ate breakfast with us three mornings a week, but on Mondays and Thursdays, his surgery days, he left the house before we were out of bed. Mom was always up to make him breakfast and see him off. Mary and I came home for lunch, which meant Mom had to have a meal ready for us the moment we arrived if we were to get back in time for the start of afternoon classes. Bob was too young for kindergarten. Billy's needs were so all-consuming that Bob spent a lot of time on his own. Mom and Dad decided to send him to a private nursery school, but that meant driving him there and picking him up. Mom tried to time trips to the grocery store for when she figured Billy would be least likely to spit up — and adjusted when he spat up anyway. A cleaner came to the house once a week, but Mom did all the rest: the cooking, the dishes, the meal planning, the shopping, the homework supervision, the laundry. And the laundry alone was, as she put it, "horrendous."

More and more, she found herself trapped. So did Dad, and he, especially, resented it. Dad worked hard and provided well for his family and, typical of men of his generation, thought his wishes, needs, and desires should come first. He loved his social life — dinners out, bridge games, parties, dances, events at the golf club, curling club, and ski club — and wanted Mom with him. But most of that fell by the wayside.

Finding a babysitter was difficult; most nights, Mom was too worn out to even think of going out, and too exhausted to enjoy herself when she did.

Mom and Dad decided to find someone to help with the house-work. They hired Esme, a domestic worker from Jamaica, as a live-in maid. This eased Mom's workload but brought complications of its own. Suddenly, the big new house felt crowded: four bedrooms had seemed like a lot when they built it, but now seven people lived in them. Mary and I shared the double room at the end of the hall. I think Bob had his own room, and Bill moved into our parents' room. Esme had her own room, but no privacy beyond that. The kids and Esme all shared one bathroom; the ensuite bathroom in our parents' room was theirs alone. Mom knew how to run a house, but managing a maid wasn't something working-class North Bay girls learned to do in the midst of the Depression. In theory, Esme's job was to take on the household chores, keep an eye on Bill, and free Mom to spend more time with Mary, Bob, and me. But all too often, it was Esme who ended up taking care of us while Mom took care of Bill. Esme left for Toronto after a short time and another live-in — Nelly, from the Netherlands — moved in. Nelly lived with us for a few months before moving out to get married but came to our house three days a week after that. I can still count to ten in Dutch, thanks to her.

As the months went by and Billy showed no signs of getting better, Mom and Dad again took up the question of what to do with him. Dad had accepted the necessity of bringing Billy home as a newborn, though he never saw that as a permanent move. The only question, in his mind, wasn't whether to admit Billy to the Ontario Hospital School at Smiths Falls but when. Mom resisted. But a brief and seemingly insignificant incident between Billy and Mary in the fall of 1958 — an encounter I doubt any of us would have remembered if Mom hadn't told us about it time and again over the years — settled the issue. One day, after church, Billy ran to hug Mary and "spurted," as Mom put it, "all over the front of her dress. From then on she more or less avoided him — understandably."[8] If the rest of us were starting to develop an aversion to Billy, then that was the sign that it was time for him to go. Dad and Mom again called

Harold Frank, the superintendent at the Ontario Hospital School. This time, Dr. Frank told them to get started on admitting Billy.

It's funny how small incidents become family legends. Mary's ruined dress was pinpointed, inside the family and out, as the incident that precipitated Bill's banishment from home. But I always had trouble believing it was such a big deal for the rest of us kids, or so critical as to be decisive. None of us liked Billy's vomiting. I know I complained, especially when he vomited on the toys or the floor. I never wore shoes inside the house — or anywhere else if I could get away with it — and the repulsive sensation of stepping in Billy's slippery goo stays with me to this day. But it was also part of who he was, just like his goofy dance in the crib, his roars of laughter at the *fa la la la la* in "Deck the Halls," his blissful smile when cuddling with Mom in the big chair in the den. I can't imagine that Mary's attitude toward Billy turned on a dime, or that our parents simultaneously or independently concluded that *this* soiled dress was the last straw.

My guess is that, at some point well before this particular Sunday, my parents had come to an agreement. They would keep Bill at home until the other children began to turn against him. That they assumed we would do so seems hard to grasp — current research suggests many siblings react positively to having a sister or brother with disabilities[9] — but it was in line with everything the experts were telling them. When Mary started avoiding Bill, I think Mom simply gave in to the inevitable. The medical establishment, the government, her friends, the pediatrician, and the other adults in the family, especially Dad and Nana, believed that sending him to an institution was the best option for everyone. If they kept Bill at home, she feared, one by one the rest of us would turn against him.

She also feared that, as Bill grew older, he would be increasingly isolated — not just in the family but in the community, too. He couldn't go to the neighbourhood public school like the rest of us; Ontario had allowed auxiliary classes for what the province categorized as feeble-minded children since the early 1900s, but only for those with IQs of

50 or higher. In the early 1950s, the province gave small grants to parent groups to run classes for kids with IQs below 50, and Bill might have been able to go to one of those.[10] But then Mom would have had to do the work of finding a class that would take him and volunteer to help run it, and the last thing she needed was more work. Even if she should find a school, she knew he wouldn't be able to join the Cub Scouts, or take swimming lessons, or skiing lessons, or join city recreation programs. Mom and Dad could see no future for him in Ottawa beyond endless days at home. If Bill's future looked grim, theirs wasn't looking too rosy, either. They wanted to raise their children, send them off into the world, and then enjoy the freedom they worked so hard to earn. But how could they do that and take care of an adult son with a significant intellectual handicap, a son with a toddler's mind in a grown man's body?

Above all, though, by the fall of 1958, I think Mom was just plain tired — tired of the mountains of laundry, the smell of vomit everywhere she turned, the guilt she felt because the least able of her four children occupied the bulk of her time. She had come to believe that, no matter what she did for her family, it wasn't enough. And with Bill at home, it might never be enough.

In early October, a month after Bill's second birthday, Mom and Dad drove to Smiths Falls to visit the institution and meet with the superintendent, Dr. Frank. A few days later, Dad sent him a letter asking for the admission documents. He added, "I want to thank you very much for your kindness when we saw you last week. I think you have helped a great deal in reassuring both my Wife and myself that we have done the right thing."[11] They began the formal process of admitting Bill to the institution in November. They found two medical experts to sign forms certifying that their youngest son was "a mentally defective patient." One of them, their friend and family pediatrician Fred Jeffrey, described Bill as unable to speak, "docile but inattentive — does not obey simple commands — walks with awkward gait." He added, "Information from mother — happy but unable to care for himself in any way."

Mom had the task of filling out the longest form, a three-page "mentally defective patient's history." The medical part was pretty straightforward. She reported that he'd had pneumonia and chicken pox, and had been immunized against diphtheria, whooping cough, smallpox, and tetanus. He'd had no serious accidents. He needed diapers at night. He could not dress himself. He slept well. Strangely, she did not mention his vomiting. In response to a question asking whether he'd had any feeding difficulties in the first two years, she wrote, "no."

Some of the other questions, however, must have made her cringe.

> Question 14. Are Father and Mother blood relations?
> Question 15. Have any relatives been mentally ill,
>   feeble-minded, epileptic, neurotic, eccentric? Give
>   particulars....
> Question 20: Moral History
>   (a) Is there a history of petty thieving or stealing?
>   (b) Does the patient do injury to himself?
>   (c) Is patient cruel to people or animals?
>   (d) Is patient a fire-setter?
>   (e) Describe patient's sex interests and experiences, if any.

Questions like these appeared to be aimed at finding out what was wrong with the family that produced the child being admitted. I'm sure she found them troubling. Another question asked whether the prospective patient was "quarrelsome, quick or violent tempered, suggestible, stubborn, seclusive, suspicious, obedient, etc." Mom's response, penned in her beautiful and clear cursive script, was terse: "Very happy and cheerful."

The final part of the form asked for the name of the responsible person for the institution to contact. On any official form having to do with the children, Mom always wrote "Dr. and Mrs. D.D. McKercher." This time, however, she wrote "Dr. D.D. McKercher." Dad's name. Just his. I can't help but wonder whether this was a final, small, futile act of resistance, a way of telling the institution — and her husband — that she had given in to his wishes and was washing her hands of any further responsibility. I suspect it was, and it breaks my heart.

The paperwork was sent and processed. Mom and Dad received a note from the institution in early December setting Bill's admission for Wednesday, February 18, 1959. This means Mom and Dad knew that the Christmas of 1958 would be Bill's last with us. The rest of us did not. The holidays must have been especially difficult for my parents that year. I have no memories of them.

Mom and Dad still had one bit of unfinished business to tend to before moving Billy to Smiths Falls: he had still not been baptized. They called the Reverend Norman Coll, the Parkdale United Church minister who had baptized the rest of us, and on a sunny, winter Wednesday afternoon — February 11, 1959 — Reverend Coll came to the house and baptized Bill. My parents made an occasion of it. I can't recall who else was there, but I know there was a small party. Nana came, of course, and a few of our parents' close friends, I think. We had tea and finger sandwiches, cookies, and desserts. Mary and I both remember it as a nice day. One week later, Billy was gone. He never came back.

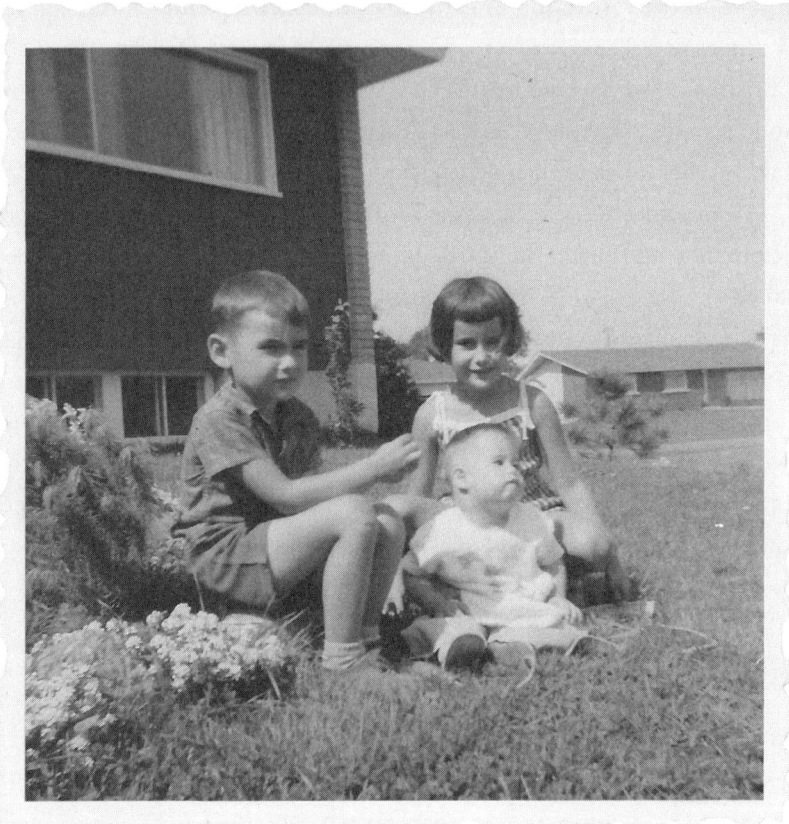

Social attitudes toward people like Bill—shown here in the family backyard
with Bob and me the summer before his move—were still pretty negative in
the 1950s. The conventional wisdom was that people with Down syndrome
were defective and had nothing to offer to the rest of us.

Chapter 3

"HOSPITALS FOR **MENTAL DEFECTIVES**"

The Ontario Hospital School at Smiths Falls, where my parents left Bill on that winter day in 1959, was one of the newest and largest facilities of its kind in North America. Its solid, brown facade conveyed an air of conservative modernity. Nothing about it was edgy or innovative. And nothing hinted at the century of hope, fear, and conflict that had given birth to institutions like it.

Until the early nineteenth century, western Europeans viewed intellectual disability as a hopeless affliction. People with these disabilities were considered uneducable. A feral child known as the Wild Boy of Aveyron, who spent years living on his own in the forests of rural France, helped change that view. No one knew who he was or where he came from, and those who took care of the boy after they captured him described him as "equally wild, impatient of restraint, and capricious in his temper."[1] They wondered whether he was a child with a disability or a *sauvage*, a human living in the original state in nature. Jean Marc Gaspard Itard, a young Parisian doctor who eventually took him in, figured the child was about twelve and had been alone in the woods for about seven years, long enough to have forgotten anything he might have known about human society. Itard was already making a name for himself educating people who were deaf, and saw this child as an opportunity to expand his skills and reputation. He named the boy Victor, and set out to teach him how to speak, read, write, and generally behave in polite society. Itard's book describing Victor's education, published in English as *An Historical*

Account of the Development and Education of A Savage Man, became a case study in the Enlightenment debate over the essential nature of humanity, the characteristics that separate people from animals, and the influence of nature versus nurture.

In the five or six years Victor lived with Itard, the boy made some progress in learning how to live with other people, but his communication skills never caught up with those of others his age. He understood what people said to him but never learned to speak, and he learned how to write just two phrases. Contemporary physicians concluded he had an intellectual disability of some sort. Modern scholars who have studied the case suspect autism.[2] Nonetheless, the fact Victor made as much progress as he did intrigued educators and doctors. If a child as intellectually and morally deprived as Victor could learn, even a little, then perhaps there was hope for other children with disabilities.

Itard's work inspired new ways of diagnosing intellectual and linguistic disabilities and new methods of instruction. Its impact spread far beyond France, and formed part of a set of intertwined beliefs about children with disabilities that characterized the middle years of the nineteenth century in Europe and North America. One strand was the Christian ideal that people have a duty to help the less fortunate, and who could be less fortunate than children with intellectual impairments? A second was what the US historians Peter Tyor and Leland Bell call "the perfectionist faith" of social reformers, who saw no limit to human potential, "no barrier that could not be overcome with the proper application of faith, hard work and knowledge."[3] These social reformers believed society could do better than relegate people like Victor to almshouses, lunatic asylums, or jails. Education was the key. By the 1840s, according to David Wright of McGill University, the mantra "the idiot could be educated" echoed across Europe and over the Atlantic to North America.[4] The enthusiasm to teach those with disabilities also had a moral dimension. The reform movement found it impossible to believe that God would create children with glaring imperfections for no good reason. Human failure, or a violation of some natural or divine law, had to have played a role in why those children existed. As the pioneering Massachusetts educator Samuel G. Howe put it, "where there was so much suffering, there must have been sin."[5] Correcting that sin and eliminating the conditions that led to it mattered to everyone. Howe argued further that "an ignorant vicious or suffering class is a disturbing force in society . . . it must be removed or there can never be order."[6]

"Boarding schools for idiots," as Howe and others called them, began to crop up across the United States in the middle of the nineteenth century as experiments in training and educating children with intellectual disabilities. It was an exciting, challenging prospect. Students, teachers, and administrators were starting from scratch, drawing on philosophical and educational theories that had been developed mainly in Europe and then transplanted to the United States. These new institutions enthusiastically pursued the goal of preparing these children to find a proper and meaningful place in society. Some schools even promised the damaged child could be cured.

Compared to the massive hospital school where my brother grew up, these early boarding schools sound idyllic.

One of the first in the United States opened in Barre, Massachusetts, in 1848, at the private home of Dr. Hervey.B. Wilbur, who would later become medical superintendent of the New York State Asylum for Idiots in Syracuse, New York. Other schools, some publicly funded and some entirely private, cropped up in New York, Pennsylvania, Massachusetts, and elsewhere in the country, generally in cities and often in state capitals. The schools brought children in at a young age, pushed them to develop to their full potential, and then sent them home when they reached a maximum age, typically sixteen. Once back in their communities, the children would, presumably, live full and rich lives. The schools generally selected their students carefully, rejecting those who were too seriously impaired, too intractable, too old, or too impoverished in other ways. Many admitted children on probation: those who showed promise could stay; those who did not, or who for any number of reasons didn't seem to be a good fit for the school, were sent home. The school would diagnose a student's particular handicaps or deficits, then work to fix them. This meant the schools had to be small and richly staffed, with lots and lots of contact between students and faculty.

Like other boarding schools, the "boarding schools for idiots" demanded—and enforced—discipline. According to Tyor and Bell, the teachers asserted their authority over the students, "generally by force of personality but by physical means if necessary."[7] New students who were noisy or rowdy were quickly instructed on how to be quiet and behave. Most schools, though, forbade corporal punishment. Instead, the schools modelled themselves after the large, Victorian-era family under the paternalistic control of a father figure, usually known as the superintendent. This arrangement appealed to both the families of the students and to the general public.

The schools shared another feature with other schools: long summer vacations. Students went home for up to two months at the end of the school year. Their families, not the schools, were to be the permanent fixtures in the lives of these children, so time spent at home to preserve the family bond was essential. Summer vacations gave the staff, who worked very long hours—six days a week during the school year—a break. The long summer vacations also cemented the purpose and identity of the schools as educational institutions, rather than places for life-long care.

The schools quickly proved popular with families, politicians, and the public. Without doubt, they offered a wonderful opportunity for a number of upper- or middle-class children with mild or moderate intellectual impairments. As Tyor and Bell put it, "a few select students, a dedicated and vigorous staff committed to educating pupils, parents and the public, along with a receptive and supportive community, created a setting, a unique educational milieu, which established a high quality of care and concern for retarded children."[8]

Almost none of these characteristics survived into the twentieth century.

—

In Britain, John Langdon Down was part of a group of reformers and educators who were pursuing the same goals as the Americans. Historian Deborah Cohen, in a book on shame and secrecy in Britain, writes that, in England, the idea that "idiots could be educated, even cured" was "Victorian medical science's equivalent of the telegraph—proof that the limits of human achievement had hardly been tapped."[9]

Down became medical superintendent of the fledgling Earlswood Asylum for Idiots in London in 1855, and it was while he was there that Down wrote his famous 1866 essay, "Observations on an Ethnic Classification of Idiots"[10] It was—and is—a remarkable analysis of the condition we now call Down syndrome. Down knew there were dozens of ways children could become intellectually impaired, but some forms cannot be explained by medical malpractice, disease, or accident. The people he called "Mongolians" are simply born that way: "They are always congenital idiots and never result from accidents after uterine life."[11]

Because this particular disability accounted for one in ten of his Earlswood patients, Down was able to study those with it both as individuals and as a group. He provided detailed physical descriptions of the condition, from the shape of faces and eyes to the fact so many suffer from weak chests. He also offered a general personality profile. He could have been describing my brother when he wrote that people with this disability "have considerable power of imitation, even bordering on being mimics. They are humorous and a lively sense of the ridiculous often colours their mimicry." Significantly, Down wrote, "this faculty of imitation can be cultivated to a very great extent and a practical direction given to the results obtained." He also observed that, although they have thick and roughened tongues, children with the disability could learn to speak. "The speech is thick and indistinct, but may be improved very greatly by a well-directed scheme of tongue gymnastics," he wrote. He also thought that training could help with physical coordination and the ability to manipulate objects: "The improvement which training effects in them is greatly in excess of what would be predicted if one did not know the characteristics of the type," he observed. At the same time, however, Down noted that the life expectancy of these people was far below average, "and the tendency is to the tuberculosis, which I believe to be the hereditary origin of the degeneracy." He was off-base there — tuberculosis has nothing to do with Down syndrome. Nonetheless, Down's essay not only describes the disability, but establishes the foundational principle of his professional life: people with intellectual disabilities can learn, and they can learn more than the rest of society expected.

As Down's reputation grew, he clashed with the Earlswood board several times, and eventually resigned. He and his wife, Mary, who had been an active volunteer at Earlswood, decided to create their own institution in a suburb southwest of London. Normansfield — they named it after their lawyer — was just the kind of place where Down could pursue his theories of education without having to answer to a board. The facility began as a family enterprise, and turned into a dynasty. It was registered in Mary Down's name; John was the medical superintendent. After John died in 1896, his sons Reginald and Percy took over and his grandson Norman became deputy medical superintendent in 1946, staying on as superintendent when Normansfield became part of the UK National Health Service in 1951. Norman retired in 1970.

Normansfield opened in 1868, in a family-style home in a large park. Its first residents were about twenty people with a variety of intellectual disabilities. Advertised as offering "home and education for the backward and feebleminded," Normansfield was beautifully furnished.[12] Handsome new buildings were added to the property as the school expanded. By 1892, it had two hundred residents. Normansfield had lots of staff, forty acres of manicured lawns and gardens, and elegant reception areas. All residents learned "life skills" such as dressing, feeding, cooking, how to use money, and how to weigh and measure things. They also learned music, dancing, and languages. Workshops taught young residents a variety of crafts; weaving was especially popular. Residents played tennis, croquet, and cricket. They posed for formal photographic portraits, some of which are posted on the website for the Langdon Down Museum of Learning Disability, which now occupies the Normansfield site. The photos of young people with Down syndrome are striking. One shows a young woman with stylishly curled hair and a velvet gown, leaning casually on a desk. In another, a girl in a less formal frock is reading a book. A young man, photographed in profile while seated, has the bearing of a country squire.[13] These are classic Victorian poses, carefully composed to show the trappings of a cultured and prosperous life. They run directly counter to the image of Down syndrome my parents had a century later, and to the photographs—basically mug shots—that my brother's institutional caretakers took of him.

Normansfield gave high priority to entertainment, in addition to education. Down built a beautiful Gothic theatre that was also used for Sunday services, and one of the main buildings held a huge playroom for the younger students. Eventually, the facility expanded to include a farm and kitchen garden. The most posh US schools looked almost spartan by comparison.

The vast majority of young people admitted to Normansfield came from well-off families. It cost one hundred and fifty guineas a year to send a child there, roughly the same fee as tuition at Britain's best schools.[14] The students were expected to stay in residence for five to seven years, then return home. They typically ranged in age from eight to sixteen, though some were younger. Deborah Cohen's book describes one resident, Lucy Gardner, who was born in 1878 and moved into Normansfield at the age of five: "Lucy brought with her trunks full of pretty clothes, a wardrobe that her anxious mother regularly replenished with deliveries of frocks, bonnets, stockings, sachets, brushes, comb-bags and sashes." Like students in the US schools, Lucy and her fellow students visited home often, and often received visitors from home. On school holidays, she went to garden parties and teas; while she was at school, her family and friends asked about her. Lucy stayed at Normansfield for four years then went home to her family, who "delightedly pronounced her much improved."[15]

In addition to their talents as educators, the Downs were skilled in generating good publicity. "Pupils who came to Normansfield unable to say more than a few words, the newspapers reported, had learned to multiply seventeen and twenty-four, to sing hymns and decline Latin nouns," Cohen writes. "On the lawn, fashionably dressed young ladies, all 'afflicted with idiocy in varying degrees,' played croquet, while in the theatre younger children performed in musical recitals. Imposing from the outside, light and airy in its interior, Normansfield called to mind a well-endowed school, not a hospital."[16]

—

While the French, Americans, and English pushed ahead with experiments in how to educate, train, and socialize people with intellectual disabilities, Canada was still trying to get them out of lunatic asylums. Mind you, the lunatic asylums were probably an improvement on the other place that commonly warehoused these people in Canada, the county jail. But, clearly, the Canadian colonies lagged far behind their colonial masters, their neighbours to the south, and much of Western Europe.

In *From Asylum to Welfare*, the definitive history of Ontario's approach towards people with intellectual disabilities, Harvey G. Simmons notes that people with intellectual disabilities were among the very first patients at the brand-new Provincial Lunatic Asylum that opened in Toronto in 1841, despite the fact that the institution's governors did not want them there.[17] The authorities saw them as an obstacle to the treatment of people with psychiatric disorders. But the law included intellectual disability as a form of lunacy, and many doctors were happy to certify people with disabilities as insane. Certification was not simply a matter of identifying a problem; it was also a way to get rid of troublemakers. Sending them to the provincial hospital solved one group's problem by turning it into someone else's problem.

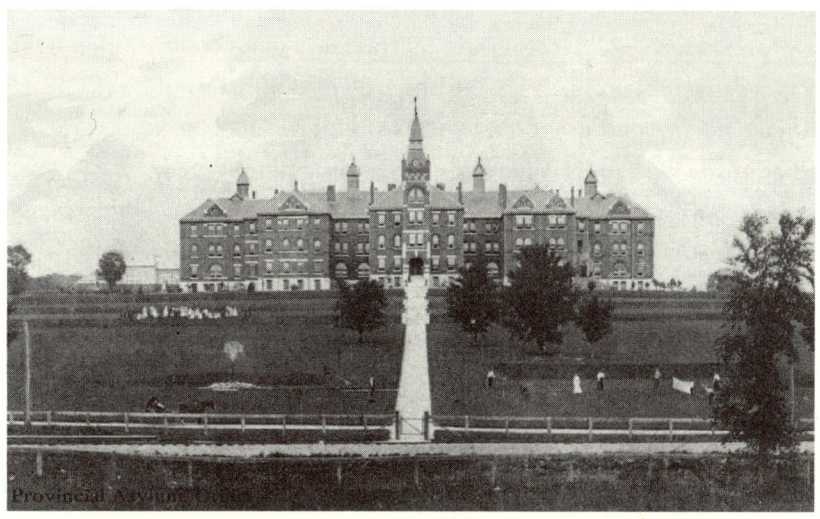

In this 1906 postcard, the Huronia institution looks like a castle, a fine and lovely asylum for people with disabilities. Life on the inside was anything but idyllic. (Courtesy of Marcel Rousseau)

Simmons says nineteenth-century Canadians with intellectual impairments followed a well-trod path, from family home to county jail to asylum to different treatment centres within the asylum. In the 1860s, many were diverted to the Orillia Branch Lunatic Asylum, which closed a few years later. In the 1870s, the Asylum for Adult Idiots in London, Ontario, opened on the grounds of the new London Asylum for the Insane. This was created as a separate residential facility, housing people who could not survive in the wider world. The average age of the first residents was twenty-two.

Some Canadian reformers, following what was going on elsewhere, promoted the idea of schools for children with intellectual disabilities. John Langmuir, who was in charge of asylums in Ontario from 1868 to 1882, was an enthusiastic fan of the experimental schools in the United States and England. In 1873, he reported that "over 50 per cent of the children trained and instructed in them are fitted to be placed in families, where they become useful and earn their own living." In Ontario, by contrast, hundreds of children "are now growing up without any training or instruction and are constantly contracting vicious habits, and in many cases dangerous propensities."[18] Running a school that would teach people independence and proper behaviour would be much more economical than throwing these people into an institution, he argued.

Ontario's first dedicated facility for people with intellectual impairments opened in Orillia in 1876. The responsibility of the same government department that oversaw charities and prisons,[19] the facility's name—in its early years, it was known variously as the Ontario Hospital for Idiots and Imbeciles and the Ontario Asylum for Idiots—reflected its purpose. It was an asylum, not a school. Its first residents came from the London Asylum for the Insane, from provincial jails, and from private homes. This last group included some children.

The institution was crowded and short of both staff and funding right from the beginning. Within two years, the youngest residents were sleeping two to a bed. A new facility, built to house 550 residents, replaced the old one in 1885. It had a massive red-brick main building, with space for classrooms on the ground floor, and dorms and sitting rooms for those who were then known as the "trainable mentally retarded"—people who might learn a skill, find work, and move back to the community—on the upper floors. Two three-storey buildings known as cottages were intended for those thought unfit for education or training.

Classrooms do not make a school, however. The province was reluctant to pay for teachers, and two years went by before the first teacher joined the staff at Orillia. And, when it finally opened, the school within the asylum was not a success. Teaching the children who lived in the institution a few songs and the basics of spelling and counting led nowhere, Simmons writes, because there was no follow-up.[20] The "high point" of the school was reached in 1896 when eight teachers were on staff, "but by 1902 the school had to be discontinued, only to be started up again the following year, but this time with two teachers," Simmons writes.[21] By then the pattern had been set: its goal was to provide care and treatment—which might include skills training—to people who, for any number of reasons, were seen to need it. The rich who wanted to send their children to private boarding schools in the United States or United Kingdom could do so, but for the rest of people in Ontario, the institution at Orillia was the only option.

Eventually, as more and more children moved into the institution, the Orillia facility expanded its classrooms. The institution's name was changed in the 1920s to the Ontario Hospital. In the 1930s it became the responsibility of the new health and public works departments and the name changed again, this time to the Ontario Hospital School. The name change was to reflect both its changing population and its broader purpose, but that purpose was a hybrid one, not single-purpose like a boarding school.

Ironically, the Ontario approach turned out to be at the forefront of the next phase of care.

The foundational principles behind the US boarding schools of the mid-nineteenth century held for about twenty years. But, by the waning years of the century, their moment was over for a number of reasons. For one, the schools did not reach their hoped-for goals. "The early estimates of the number of retarded who could be returned as self-supporting to the community were far too high," Tyor and Bell write.[22] Children, when first entering the schools, would develop quickly — largely because they were children, growing and responding to the intense and supportive educational environment of the school. The superintendents at the time believed the children would continue to make progress at the same rate but, by the 1870s, those in charge realized they had been overly optimistic. The Pennsylvania Training School for Idiotic and Feeble-Minded Children reported that, of five hundred people who had gone through schooling there, only eighty-one — a little over 15 per cent — were capable of supporting themselves fully when they finished school. Another 140 were capable of earning some portion of their expenses, and 118 were judged able to perform small services and chores. Almost one-third of the former students, however, remained "hopelessly dependent," despite years of schooling. Drawing on records from his own institution, the superintendent extrapolated the financial condition of the roughly thirty-five hundred people with intellectual disabilities then living in Pennsylvania. His conclusion was grim: about seven hundred came from families who could support them fully, and another 650 from families who could provide partial support. Roughly sixteen hundred came from families who were poor but didn't want to put their relatives in public almshouses, and 570 were already living in the almshouse.[23] Given that the schools had been founded in part to keep people out of these kinds of places, this was a disappointing—and disturbing—result.

To a degree, the schools were the victims of their own success. The early, positive results led to pressure to take in more and more students. The schools expanded and grew, but, every time they did, the demand outstripped the supply of spaces. At the same time, schools were facing pressure to expand their mandates by taking in older people, including young adults and people with severe disabilities or multiple disabilities who needed long-term care more than education. And, as students came to reach the age of sixteen or seventeen, the authorities realized that many of them had no place to go. The age for students to leave began to creep up. Summer vacations back home—once seen as critical to keeping students in touch with the communities that would eventually be their homes—began to disappear amid a growing realization that many students would never be at home in their communities. More and more, the people who ran the schools and the other social institutions that took care of people with intellectual disabilities began to talk about the need for a different kind of institution—an asylum, which would provide long-term housing, work, and care for adults.

The movement from boarding school to asylum proceeded in stages.

An early step was a form of in-house segregation that divided the resident body into groups based on how the people running the schools assessed their capabilities. Authorities feared that the well-trained or advanced students would relapse if they were kept in the same classrooms as the less able students. This led to a change in the physical layout of the schools, with the construction of separate buildings for the various groups. Hospital wings were erected for residents who were confined to

bed, or in some cases to cribs, and completely unable to care for themselves.

Many of the early schools were in urban areas or on large tracts of
suburban land, like Normansfield in England. The newer asylums tended
to be in the countryside, built as more or less self-contained villages.
In return for their care, the residents worked to keep the institution
going. The men worked in the fields, or made brooms, mats, brushes,
or cane-bottom chairs, while the women laboured in the kitchens or
the laundry, or sewed linens and clothing. Some residents were assigned
to the hospital wing to care for residents with more severe disabilities.
Putting the residents to work meant the institution could reduce the
number of paid workers needed to run the facility, and selling some of
the products of their labour—the chairs, the linens, the brooms, the farm
produce—would bring in income, generate good publicity, and possibly
inspire generous donations. Ideally, the institution might even become
self-sufficient.

Eventually, the asylum supplanted the educational institution. The
basic mission of the "villages of the simple," as Tyor and Bell call them,[24]
was to provide people with intellectual disabilities with a safe, simple, and
protected life, away from the rest of society. Families could stay in touch,
but more and more the assumption was that residents would never leave.

—

The early reformers saw people with intellectual disabilities as God's most
fragile creatures, arriving on Earth as the result of some unknown divine
plan. As the nineteenth century came to a close, a harsher analysis came
to the fore: God didn't cause intellectual disability, people did. Gustavus
Doren, superintendent in the mid-1860s of an institution in Columbus,
Ohio, put it bluntly, not to mention biblically: "the children of men must
inherit their ills."[25] These ills, as defined at the time, ran from alcohol
abuse to excessive sexual activity, and from arduous physical or mental
labour to marriage between members of the same family. It was already
known that some forms of psychiatric illness ran in families, so it was

an easy leap for many to conclude that intellectual disability must do so as well. Scientists, policy makers, and school authorities in general became convinced that hereditary weakness was responsible for nearly all cases of intellectual disabilities. The people with the disabilities might be innocents, but their families were not. And that was a problem for everyone.

In Britain, the expansion of mandatory education in the 1870s brought a new group of students with intellectual impairments to school, mainly rural or working-class children who might have passed without notice in a society where farm or factory workers had no need for literacy. The authorities categorized them as feeble-minded. Quite quickly, intellectual deficiencies came to be seen as a social problem, and not just an individual or private problem. Authorities on both sides of the Atlantic worried about what they saw as a growing underclass of feeble-minded people, breeding like rabbits and threatening the moral and physical welfare of society. They believed feeble-mindedness was linked to poverty, crime, alcoholism, juvenile delinquency, incest, and other social ills. Feeble-minded women were especially dangerous. They had fewer inhibitions against sex, the authorities believed, and were especially fertile, passing on their feeble-mindedness to their large broods of children. "The feeble-minded are a parasitic, predatory class, never capable of self-support or of managing their own affairs. The great majority become public charges in some form. They cause unutterable sorrow at home and a menace and danger to the community," asserted the head of the Massachusetts School for the Feeble-Minded, Walter E. Fernald. "Every feeble-minded person, especially the high-grade imbecile, is a potential criminal."[26] Fernald believed people with intellectual disabilities should be sent for care to custodial institutions — in other words, locked up without trial — and that some should be sterilized in hopes of eliminating the next generation. In Britain, writes Deborah Cohen, "the weak in intellect had, by the turn of the century, become a danger — even *the* danger facing the nation."[27]

Early sociological studies of families like the Jukes of New York

State, purporting to show that both feeble-mindedness and criminality ran in families, gave what the British sociologist Pauline Morris calls "a scientific *imprimatur* to the belief that mental defect was, *and could only be*, inherited."[28] If this was so, and if defectives were allowed to marry and procreate in large numbers, authorities believed the result would be the degradation of the human species. According to Cohen, "By 1901, when the new category of feeble-minded was included in the census, statisticians discovered 133,000 mental defectives in Britain, a figure that bore out the most dire predictions. Writing in the *British Medical Journal* that same year, the physician W.H. Dickinson warned that Britain's future 'depended largely on the stamping out of feeble-mindedness.'"[29]

This added a new twist to the rationale for asylums for people with intellectual disabilities. If these people needed protection from the rest of society, the reverse also held true. Society needed protection from them.

John Langdon Down rejected simplistic causes of intellectual disability. He believed that, in the vast majority of cases, the cause was unknown. His son Reginald, who ran Normansfield after his father's death and was a prominent member of the Eugenics Society, took a harder line. The eugenicists saw two ways to solve the problem of intellectual disabilities: one was to encourage what they saw as the "right" kind of people to have children; the other was to stop the "wrong" kind of people—and especially, the feeble-minded—from breeding. And the best way to achieve this goal was compulsory institutionalization, where residents would be segregated by sex and, in many cases, sterilized. Cohen notes that Reginald Langdon-Down personally advocated for the sterilization of the mentally unfit.[30]

This shift in how experts thought about how to care for those with intellectual disability was reflected in concrete changes to social policy. Asylums were still seen as the answer, but the goal of asylums was now to keep the feeble-minded away from the healthy population, not just to care for them humanely. In 1914, the Ontario government appointed an influential proponent of eugenics, Dr. Helen MacMurchy,[31] as provincial inspector of the feeble-minded, a job she held for five years. MacMurchy argued that "abnormal" children should be sent as early as possible to the asylum in Orillia. The asylum's main value, in her view, was as a means to prevent feeble-minded children from growing up to be the parents of more feeble-minded children. MacMurchy also advocated for the compulsory sterilization of women judged unfit to bear children.[32] Ontario resisted passing a law on forced sterilization for the purpose of eugenics, although two other Canadian provinces and thirty-three states in the United States did enact this kind of legislation during this time period. But the Ontario government encouraged sterilization for women at Orillia and at a new facility in Cobourg, east of Toronto, which opened in 1920 as a women's psychiatric hospital. By 1938, women labelled as having intellectual disabilities accounted for almost two-thirds of the 461 residents in the Cobourg facility, many of whom had been sent there simply because they had become pregnant. A provincial royal commission on the Mental Health Act proposed that if those women agreed to be sterilized, they could be released. "While they would still be a sex problem in the community they would not be the same problem," the commission concluded.[33]

The eugenics movement was inextricably linked not just to intellect but to race as well. In the United States, working-class African American women were the main target of compulsory sterilization. Civil rights leader Fannie Lou Hamer popularized the term "Mississippi appendectomy" to refer to sterilization operations done on African American women without their consent or knowledge. She had undergone one of these herself during surgery to remove a tumour in 1961.[34] In Canada, Indigenous women—who were also more likely to be diagnosed as mentally defective —were targets.[35] Nazi Germany, of course, took the practice of eugenics the furthest, using forced sterilization, breeding programs, euthanasia campaigns, and genocide as tools to create a so-called master race and suppress or eliminate everyone else. People with intellectual disabilities were high on the Nazi lists for extermination.

As the eugenics movement reached its peak in the 1920s and 1930s, the charge of a hereditary taint could have a devastating effect on an entire family. The problem was no longer simply one of stopping the feeble-minded from propagating: "Now, the science of heredity had revealed that even those seemingly of normal intelligence could be 'carriers' for imbecility; one idiot in the family was an indictment of all," Cohen writes. Especially for middle-class professionals, "to have a mentally deficient child was to face personal and professional humiliation."[36] According to the American historian James W. Trent, "to have a defective in the family was to be associated with vice, immorality, failure, bad blood, and stupidity."[37] These children were a mark of shame, and the only remedy was to hide them away. Doctors advised more and more parents to cut their losses by sending the children to institutions.

This was the era in which my parents grew up, and Cohen's account resonates with what I know about my own family. My parents both came from families that were intolerant of difference and quick to judge. After my father's Aunt Annie died, we found among her belongings a fat, illustrated book on the so-called science of eugenics. When my brother Bill was born, Annie and her older sister, Ella, blamed my mother. No one on her side of the family, Ella told my McKercher cousins, had ever produced such a child. The King family must have "tainted blood," she said. Bessie, my grandmother, was among the first to suggest sending Bill to an institution. I am sure Ella and Annie agreed.

—

The popular conception people have of the provincial hospital school today is that it was a home and training centre for children with intellectual disabilities. But, from the outset, these institutions were always much more than that. The oldest one in Ontario, at Orillia, housed adults as well as children, including senile elderly people, people with multiple handicaps, and people with advanced syphilis. It took in orphans or abandoned children who had nowhere else to go, children who had failed to thrive in foster care, young people who had trouble finding work, and pregnant women with no one to support them. Resident labour—on the farm, in the laundry and kitchen, in building cleaning and maintenance, or tending to other patients—kept staffing costs to a minimum. Most people admitted under the guise of social welfare were assessed as having "mild" intellectual impairments, the basic requirement for a spot in the institution. However, their most common shared characteristic, no matter what their physical or intellectual condition, was poverty.[38]

In a 2013 book, author Thelma Wheatley describes one Toronto family's experience with the Orillia institution from 1900 to 1960.[39] Several members of the family, all of them poor and undereducated, had been sent there over that time, and the portrait of the institution she paints is horrifying: massive wards overseen at night by a single attendant; frequent rapes of both boys and girls; humiliating admission rituals; girls forced to provide nursing care for elderly, incontinent, and senile women; boys forced to shovel coal in unsafe conditions; menstrual pads handed out, collected, and counted by staff to track whether a girl got pregnant; cruel punishments, such as wrapping children in cold, wet sheets for disobeying the rules; casual violence handed out in the name of discipline; strict controls on when or whether a parent could visit; filth everywhere. But no matter how many people the province admitted to the hospital school, there was constant pressure to take in more. The institution was the anchor for a ragtag social safety net of municipal houses of refuge, special refuges for women, the hospital in Cobourg for delinquent girls, hostels run by churches or other charitable groups, and children's welfare organizations, all with paths that led to or from Orillia.

In the midst of a hard-fought Ontario election campaign in 1934, the governing Conservatives decided it was time for a second large institution, and it selected Smiths Falls, a faithfully Conservative eastern Ontario town suffering from high unemployment, as the site for it. Front-page stories in the *Smiths Falls Record News* of May 17 and May 24, 1934, anticipated an imminent announcement from the health minister that the new institution, modelled after the one at Orillia, would go up on a farm north of town. Plans called for a three-storey brick building at the centre of a large block that would include a powerhouse, nurses' residence, and other structures. The facility, with an initial cost of $1 million, would house seven hundred people. A subhead on the May 17 story pointed out that construction would provide work for "hundreds of local men."[40]

The formal announcement of the facility didn't come until mid-June, at the very end of the provincial election campaign.[41] Days later, a Liberal landslide threw the Conservatives out of power and the plans for the institution went down with the government. Public finance records show that Ontario spent roughly $47,500 on the project in 1934 and $5,000 in the first half of 1935. After that, the money dried up.[42]

When the Conservatives returned to power after the Second World War, the project was put back on track. In July of 1946, the *Record News* reported that the province was again assembling land, this time south of town, for a $2 million "provincial mental institution."[43] A month later, the province officially announced that the institution, now referred to by the newspaper as an "eastern hospital for mental defectives," would occupy three hundred acres of farmland overlooking the Rideau River.[44] The lengthy front-page story said preliminary construction would start with a minimum of delay.

The article paid little attention to the institution itself, concentrating instead on why Smiths Falls was a good choice for the facility. The town was a crossroads for several railroad lines, which would make it easier for families to visit, and the site itself was beautiful: "In point of natural scenic beauty few locations in Ontario afford a more pleasing prospect," according to the *Record News*. It had excellent drainage for storm runoff and for the operation of a modern sewage plant to serve the hospital. The site's proximity to the town would "aid staff housing problems," and future staff could also take advantage of "excellent shopping facilities" and the possibility of participating "in the social and community activities of a sizable town." As for the "mental defectives" who would live in the institution, the newspaper noted that much of the land was already under cultivation and more could be turned into farm plots and gardens, "thus affording valuable occupation for patients over a number of years."

The description is fascinating for what it highlights, what it leaves out, and what it takes for granted. Although the facility at Orillia had been renamed as the neutral-sounding Ontario Hospital in the 1920s, the newspaper report used language from the eugenics era to describe the new facility—a "hospital for mental defectives." It's impossible to tell whether this phrase originated within the newspaper or came from government sources, but either way it reveals that pre-war attitudes about people with intellectual disabilities still held in post-war Ontario.

The province could have used the new institution as an opportunity to start fresh, learn from the experience at Orillia, and experiment with new techniques in design, care, and education. It did none of this. Two world wars and close to seventy years after the Orillia institution was founded, the twentieth-century institution simply mimicked the nineteenth-century one. Geography and architecture aside, they would be the same kind of facility.

Just how much alike were they? A critical 1971 Ontario investigation into how the province cared for people with intellectual disabilities found that the only advantage the Smiths Falls facility had over the one at Orillia was that it was "newer, easier to keep clean and less of a fire hazard."[45] Around the same time that report came out, the influential disability advocate Wolf Wolfensberger, a key figure behind the movement to bring people with intellectual disabilities out of the institutions and into the community, reflected on why newer institutions like the one at Smiths Falls followed the same patterns as the older ones. "It is interesting that when the scientific rationale on which the large, dehumanizing, segregated institutions were based was rejected...no new rationale emerged," he wrote. "It seemed as if the frenzy of the alarmist period had drained the vitality out of the professionals in the field." The people planning and running the institutions either had no new ideas or lacked the ability and energy to explore them; instead, Wolfensberger wrote, they simply kept on doing what they had done before. "When you look at the anachronistic social systems that are our older institutions today, you can only understand them if you see them as living relics coasting on the momentum of the fire of another age—like the astronomer's 'white dwarfs' (spent stars), except that they are large."[46] And *large* does not begin to describe the institution at Smiths Falls.

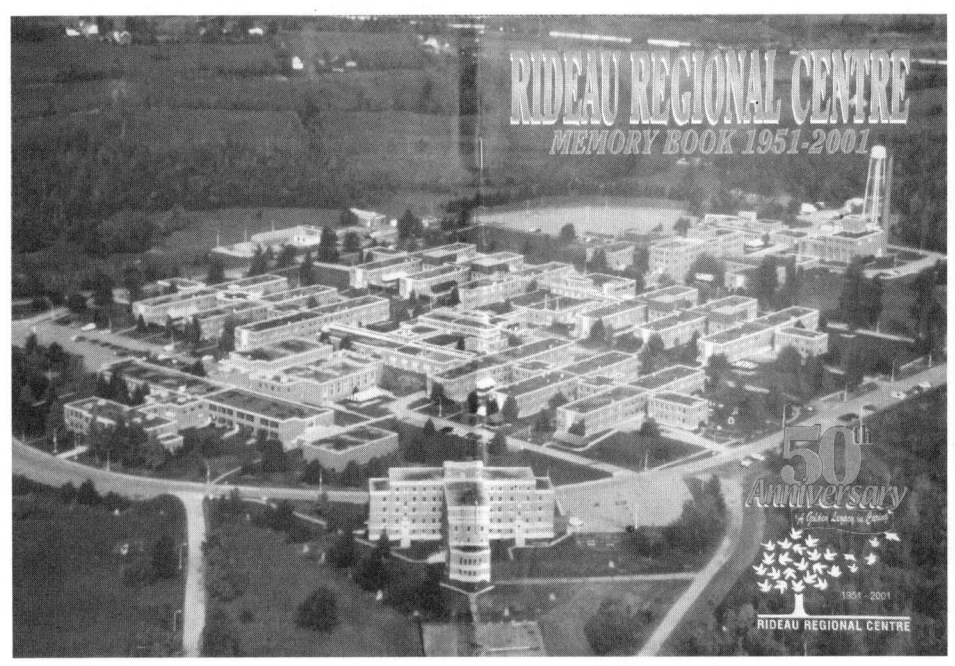

At its peak, the Rideau Regional Centre—originally the Ontario Hospital School at Smiths Falls—was so large an aerial photograph of the property filled both the front and back cover of a 2001 commemorative booklet.

Chapter 4

"PROGRESS AND HAPPINESS"

The Ontario Hospital School at Smiths Falls sat on more than four hundred acres just outside town. Construction began in the fall of 1946, with an initial budget of $14 million, and continued on and off for many, many years. The much-touted view of the Rideau River was a myth for most residents, who lived well back from the water. Staff and visitors entered the property on a long, angled driveway leading to a ring road that circled more than fifty connected buildings, totalling more than eight hundred thousand square feet of space. Most buildings were two-storey, modular, and constructed of brown brick. The residential wings—identical from the outside—branched off a central corridor that was itself more than one-third of a mile long. Smiths Falls historian Glenn J. Lockwood calls it "the largest public works project in eastern Ontario since the building of the Rideau Canal," the waterway dug in the early nineteenth century as a defence in case of war with the United States.[1] (The canal is a UNESCO World Heritage site; the institution at Smiths Falls most decidedly is not.)

When completed, the institution had five miles of corridors, more than a mile of underground tunnels, more than ten thousand doors, and twelve thousand windows. It had its own powerhouse, administration and maintenance buildings, a school wing, kitchens, bakeries, a butcher shop, some workshops, a pasteurizing room, hospital and infirmary wings, and, eventually, a swimming pool. The clinical building had hospital units, X-ray machines, operating rooms for minor surgeries, and dental offices. A fiftieth anniversary commemorative booklet published in 2001 reported that the institution's transportation department operated more than thirty vehicles. The laundry, with a staff of sixty in 1972, washed more than four and a half tonnes of clothing and linens a year. The farm had eighty acres under cultivation, plus twenty-five hundred square feet of hothouse space, and produced 433.5 tonnes of vegetables—potatoes, cabbages, lettuce, and tomatoes. From 1951 to 2001, the kitchen staff, with the help of residents, prepared more than seventy-seven million resident meals and twenty million meals for staff.[2] In just about every respect, it was a city unto itself.

The first residents were thirty men who had been living in a psychiatric hospital in Kingston. They moved into the facility in January of 1951. The women arrived in May—thirty of them, transferred from other hospitals in Ontario. Children began arriving in June, some sent by their families, others by children's aid societies. Wards for infants opened three years later, in 1954.[3]

As at Orillia, overcrowding was a problem almost from the start. In May of 1958, just seven years after the institution opened and less than a year before my brother moved in, the superintendent, Dr. Harold Frank, wrote a memo to the chief of the mental health division complaining that all the wards for males were overcrowded—four of them by 33 per cent, and the rest by 8–15 per cent. The institution's permanent bed capacity for males at that time was 960, plus fifty "transient" beds in the infirmary or in isolation. Instead, it had 1,074 male residents, with another forty on probation. "The arrangement of the wards is such, as you know, that abnormally large groups of children have to be 'corralled' into very inadequate day-room space," Frank wrote. As a result, "minor difficulties arise which are much more preventable under normal circumstances, but for which we cannot be responsible under conditions of 33 per cent overcrowding."[4] He did not specify what those minor difficulties were, but his description of children being "corralled" is chilling. This was not the first time he had complained about overcrowding: his memo says he was drawing the minister's attention to the problem "again." Over the following years, the situation would only get worse. At its peak in the mid-1960s, according to the province, 2,650 people were living there in a space designed for about two thousand.[5] This meant it was more than 25 per cent over capacity.

—

How an institution works depends in large part, Wolf Wolfensberger argues, on the problem it's meant to solve. An institution that equates intellectual disability with illness or some failure of mind or body, for example, will be called a hospital, and its director will be a physician. Its hierarchy, daily schedule, and the language it uses to describe its mission will all resemble those of a hospital. "Resident care is called nursing care; residents are called patients, and their retardation is referred to as an illness or disease," Wolfensberger explains. The process of assessing a new resident is called diagnosis and all management procedures — even education, work, and recreation — are called therapy or treatment. "Those who 'administer' such therapy (perhaps in 'doses' rather than lessons) may be called therapists." The medical model is, however, only one approach. An institution that views its residents as subhuman or as a potential threat to others will have different characteristics, such as "strong fences and window guards; locked doors; rigid segregation of the sexes; little or no use of knives and forks; unbreakable windows, dishware and furniture; staff looking at residents from protected stations rather than interacting in their midst; an open view of residents' beds, toilets, lavatories and bathrooms; prohibition of the carrying of matches, lighters and pocket knives; and rigid control and censorship over incoming and outgoing mail, parcels and telephone calls."[6]

Ontario's hospital schools shared characteristics of both models. In line with the medical model, the superintendent was a medical doctor. Residents were known as patients and lived in wards, not dormitories. Doctors, nurses, and other medical staff wore uniforms and white lab coats and ate separately from the residents they cared for, in their own cafeteria. The primary job of the people who worked on the wards was to take care of the physical needs of the patients, to make sure they were fed, dressed, cleaned, and given whatever treatment the authorities prescribed. This might include academic or practical instruction, including how to dress, use the bathroom, brush teeth, and so on. In the newer facilities like the one at Smiths Falls, hard surfaces—terrazzo floors, tiled walls, institutional chrome fixtures—allowed for easy cleaning. Though they were called hospital schools, the health department ran the school part until 1965, when the education department took over.

The white-coated medical model, however, grew out of—and on top of—the earlier model that treated people with intellectual disabilities as potentially dangerous to society. The institution at Orillia was the template, but strong remnants of that approach showed up at Smiths Falls and at the even newer Cedar Springs facility in southwestern Ontario, which opened in the early 1960s. Male and female patients lived separately, ate separately, worked separately, and had little or no casual contact with each other. Ward doors and block corridor doors were locked at all times. Residents were not allowed into the corridor unless a ward attendant went with them. In the residents' living spaces, rows of identical beds stretched from one end of the room to the other, sometimes separated by a single hard chair. There was no space for personal property, and residents weren't allowed to have personal possessions anyway; many residents wore clothing that belonged to the institution. Ward aides and attendants, who had no special qualifications when they were hired but instead took courses on the job, dressed in ways that reflected both models. The women wore uniforms like those of practical nurses. The men wore charcoal grey uniforms with black stripes on the trousers and around the cuffs of the sleeves. With rings of keys to lock and unlock the wards dangling from their belts, they looked more like prison guards than hospital workers.

Both models were inherently authoritarian, run from the top down and with residents at the bottom of the hierarchy. The people in charge of the institutions made all the decisions about day-to-day life and set all the rules. The people living in them were expected to comply or face consequences. Overcrowding and understaffing were endemic.

One former staff member's recollection of life on her ward at Smiths Falls in the early 1970s paints a vivid picture of how institutional life dehumanized the residents. In her ward, three staff members were in charge of forty-eight residents. "It was horrible," she told me. "Like living on an assembly line." For meals, the staff members had to shepherd all forty-eight to the cafeteria at once. A couple of the women in her group were known "runners" and so had to wear restraints known as Posey vests, with a staff member holding the strings. Once the staff members got the women seated and settled, one would stay with them while the other two brought trays of food. The food — "it was awful," this staff member said; "I wouldn't eat it" — disappeared in seconds. "Sometimes there'd be fights. Sometimes people choked." Then the three staff members got everybody wiped off, back on their feet, and back to the ward. A few hours later, they had to do it all over again for the next meal.

The women who lived on this ward had a shower once a week. On shower day, the staff helped all the residents undress and then lined them up. One staff member herded the women into the showers, a second was in charge of soap and shampoo, and the third helped the residents towel off. If a resident soiled herself or got dirty between showers, the ward had a slab room with a shower hose to clean them off. The residents wore institutional clothes: corduroy shorts with elastic waistbands and T-shirts, no bras, and no shoes or socks.

The former staff member also recalled that the women did not have regular menstrual periods because they were given injections of the controversial birth control drug Depo-Provera. The drug had not been approved for use as a contraceptive in Canada — that wouldn't happen until 1997 — but doctors at the Ontario institutions had already begun using it in the mid-1960s to suppress menstruation and improve "the overall hygienic circumstances for the resident, as well as her neighbours."[7] A 1981 report on the use of Depo-Provera at Smiths Falls and the other Ontario facilities noted that institutional overcrowding had been at its peak in the 1960s, and with no housekeepers assigned to wards, a drug that suppressed menstruation was "a particularly desirable management technique."[8] In the vast majority of cases where it was prescribed, no consent was obtained. Depo-Provera was given to girls as young as eleven and to women as old as fifty-one, and especially to those whose disabilities were judged to be severe or profound. At Smiths Falls, 250 women were injected with the drug in the 1960s and 1970s; other institutions also used it, though to a lesser extent. Use of Depo-Provera declined sharply by 1980, in part because of concerns about the consent issue and possible adverse health effects. However, the casual way the institutions prescribed and used Depo-Provera during the 1960s and 1970s reveals a good deal about their authoritarian nature: not only were the women on this ward dehumanized, but they were desexed as well—in most cases not for any therapeutic purpose, but simply as a way of "managing" unruly female bodies.

—

Part of my goal in taking on this project was to get a sense of what my brother Bill's day-to-day life was like in the institution at Smiths Falls. I knew this would not be easy. While scholars have studied the social policies that created the institutions and the social attitudes that shaped them, and journalists have alternately exposed abuses and offered sympathetic portraits of residents and staff, I found almost nothing from the perspective of the residents.

Occasional glimpses exist, however.

One can be found in a 1972 article by an unnamed resident of the Cedar Springs institution, in rural Blenheim near Chatham, Ontario. It appeared in the *Smiths Falls Record News* under the headline "Viewpoint: Retarded Resident Writes."[9] An editor's note at the start of the article said the resident wrote it himself and it was not edited in any manner.

When the writer arrived at the institution in the 1960s, life on the inside was difficult, harsh, and demeaning: "I always thought the staff were mean.... And I didn't even like the rules... even the privileges were strict.... On the wards we used to sit on hard chairs.... The TV we were not a loud to touch it, only the staff.... We never had good curtains.... Our beds had to be perfectly made or we practice making beds all day until we know how to do it right. We were not aloud to sit or lay down on our beds."

They also noted that life followed rigid routines and that personal possessions were discouraged: "We were never aloud to have breakfast on the ward.... We were never aloud to sleep in on Sunday morning." Bedtime was nine p.m., no exceptions: "We had to line up nice and straight.... The doors on the ward had to be locked at night.... Every night we had shoe inspection.... When we went out on a visit you had to share the things you got with the boys on the ward.... We were never aloud to have radios, watches, record players.... We were never aloud to have a razor.... We never had good clothes unless it was given to us by are parents. We were never aloud to have a coffee pot or a toaster."

Moreover, residents who smoked were "never aloud to carry a lighter or matches." Contact with female residents was strictly controlled and monitored: "The only time we were aloud to see our girlfriends was on Friday night at the dance. This place used to be runed by two or three nurses up front." During the weekdays there was little to do: "We never had instructors to teach us different jobs.... We never had a sheltered workshop.... We never had arts & crafts." The residents worked, "but we never used to get paid." Even personal grooming was subject to control: "We always had to have short hair.... We never had underarm Deodorant of our own we always had to line up and somebody would squirt us with it." The punishment for misbehaving was public humiliation: "If we got into trouble we had to wear a night gown plus we had to work on another ward."

The editor's note at the top of the column points to a 1969 Department of Health switch from a general ward system to a unit system at the three big hospital schools, which divided residents into groups and tailored programs more closely to their needs and abilities. The author of the article liked the changes: "Things are much better than they used to be to-day," he concluded. But the life he describes in his early years at Cedar Springs—years that overlapped with my brother's childhood at Smiths Falls—is dehumanizing in so many ways. The nightgown punishment was public shaming, inviting ridicule from others and at the same time warning them about what would happen when someone broke a rule. Locked wards sound like prison ranges, with residents having no freedom, no privacy, and no personal space. But the image that really makes me wince is that of the line of shirtless boys, their arms raised, waiting for a spray of deodorant. It's humiliating—and heartbreaking—no matter how you look at it. I can't help but think it's significant that the author begins his story by recalling the exact date he moved in to Cedar Springs: "On July 12, 1963 when I first came to this place I thought I would never like it here at first but after a couple of months I sort of got used to it." That was the day his life changed forever.

—

In the wake of critical media reports in 1960 about overcrowding and poor living conditions at Orillia, the province took to the airwaves to ease concerns about—and drum up public support for—the institutions. It commissioned a half-hour film, *One on Every Street*, which aired on CBC TV in April 1961.[10]

The film acknowledged that overcrowding was a significant problem at Orillia, and that some buildings were dilapidated. Yes, the film's narrator conceded, Orillia had seven hundred more residents than it should, and the waiting list to get in was huge; and yes, the institution needed more staff, including psychiatrists, psychiatric nurses, childcare specialists, social workers, physiotherapists, and teachers. Nonetheless, the film described Orillia as "a crowded but well-run community." At its core, *One on Every Street* is an idealized vision of the hospital school system, as well as an emphatic argument about why its existence served a useful purpose.

The film opens in a doctor's office, where two distraught parents have just learned that their daughter is, in the language of the day, mentally retarded. The doctor reassures them that their daughter's disability is not their fault, and that it's a common problem. One in thirty-three people — or "one on every street" — has an intellectual handicap of some sort, he says. The parents ask what they should do for their daughter. "Just what comes naturally," the doctor says. "Love her. Look after her. Some day we may have to see about putting her under the care of one of the Ontario hospital schools." The parents gasp, horrified, and ask whether the doctor means an institution. "You can call it that if you like," he says. "I prefer to think of these places as communities where a child can be happy, sometimes very useful." Ordinary people find "modern living" a little overwhelming at times, he reminds the parents. "Just think how devastating it must be for the retarded to cope with the world. Your little girl may even be happier, better off in a community which she can understand, a community where she is understood."

At this point, the film hits its main theme: hospital schools offer children with intellectual disabilities their best chance for progress and happiness. "Progress and happiness," the narrator of the documentary repeats. "These are the key words." Every child in the institution has the security and support to develop his own aptitudes: "He will study if he is able, learn to look after himself, and, most important, play, work, eat and sleep surrounded by those who understand him.... They eventually integrate so well into life at school that sometimes parents are disturbed by what seems to be a double loyalty, until they realize that this is as it should be. The school is doing a good job and the role of the parent has changed for the time being."

The bulk of the film presents images of clean, well-scrubbed, tidily dressed young people — ranging from "mildly retarded" to "severely re-tarded" — going about their daily activities. Aside from a few brief shots of the other institutions, the film concentrates on the Ontario Hospital School at Orillia. Scenes show children putting together a puzzle, marching in time to the music in a kindergarten class, and learning how to sing "Happy Birthday" in a speech therapy class. In one shot, a teenage boy takes an IQ test; in another, white-coated doctors and nurses meet with a smiling girl to assess her for admission. There are scenes of teenagers in a school classroom; young women learning cooking skills in the kitchen, working in the sewing room, and learning how to style hair in the beauty salon; young men learning to use tools in the wood shop and stitching a boot in the shoemaker's shop. The voice-over suggests that many of these "higher-functioning" youth would finish their training and, with the help of rehabilitation centres in the city, return to "normal life." Many of the children shown on screen have Down syndrome, but with rare exceptions they are not in the so-called higher-functioning groups.

Institutional life is not all about work and school, the narrator says. A segment on recreation shows girls playing basketball in the gym, young boys playing drums, triangles, tambourines, and sticks in a rhythm band, a Cub Scout meeting and a Brownies meeting. Hockey, bowling, and swimming are all part of the plan.

Only one scene shows the living conditions of adult residents at Orillia. This ward, populated by men with severe disabilities, is also the only one that is clearly in poor repair, with peeling paint and rusting pipes. It's home to "the hopeless ones," the narrator says: "One day they will have their own hospitals," but for now they live in a "community within a community," apart from the children.

Interspersed with the group scenes are close-ups of individual residents, most being tended to gently by women in crisp white nurse uniforms or specialists in lab coats. Many of these children have severe disabilities—they are unable to feed themselves, or to sit upright—and some have a combination of physical, intellectual, and psychiatric disabilities, like a young girl with a scratched face whose arms are tied to the arms of her chair. A passing nurse smiles at her and pats her gently on the hand. The narrator explains that restraints are used "in the odd case" where the resident poses a physical danger.

The film's final scene shows hundreds of young residents participating in what the narrator calls "the disciplined security of a regular Sunday service" in a large auditorium at the institution. In this scene, as in every other, the children are carefully dressed, their hair brushed and shoes shined. The boys wear dress shirts and ties, the girls wear frocks, and uniformed nurses sit among them. The choir consists of older boys in black blazers, white shirts, and black bow ties, and older girls in black blazers and white blouses, wearing identical pale pink, beaded necklaces. Church clothes are just one of many outfits the residents wear throughout the film: in other scenes they wear school uniforms, gym bloomers, grey kitchen uniforms, waitress uniforms with white aprons, and band uniforms with tall hats and gold pompoms. The clothes look reassuring—a sign of cleanliness, order, and good management. I don't ever remember seeing Bill in any kind of uniform, and the only time I saw him in a tie was when he was lying in his coffin.

Despite acknowledging the problem of overcrowding, only one quick shot, of a boys' dormitory jammed with beds, actually shows it. In the other scenes, the children are in small groups, with plenty of staff members on hand. Two women in nurses' uniforms, for example, help the seven girls working on jigsaw puzzles. In another ward, a woman working in a glassed-in nursing station keeps an eye on about ten girls in a spacious day room. The speech therapy class has six pupils; the kindergarten class, nine. Eight boys make up the rhythm band. The Cub Scout meeting has fewer than that, and the Brownie meeting has just a handful of girls. The overall impression is one of calm, orderly, and supportive supervision.

The narrated script stresses the benefits of institutional life. Some examples:

> "If the child is capable of academic training, a program is devised which will provide the best chance for those two important things: progress and happiness."

"Each child's schooling is attuned to his mental age, not his actual age, and the students are in school until they have absorbed all the knowledge they can."

"No patient is ever pushed beyond individual capacity, mental or physical."

"Accomplishments are important to retarded children. Every skill learned is a badge of honour."

"Every activity contributes to the patient's happiness and ultimately to self sufficiency and self respect."

The film ends with the minister of health, Dr. Matthew Dymond, peeking in on the church service then going to a nearby office to speak directly to the camera. He assures the audience that the government is doing its best to solve the overcrowding problem. "New buildings have been going up just as quickly as time and money have allowed," he says. "But it's not good enough. The simple solution is more staff, buildings and facilities. Not so simple, you say. Well, you're right. Every extra dollar the government spends to improve and expand these facilities must come from you, in taxes." He praises the Ontario Association for Retarded Children for its efforts in organizing community day schools and in raising public awareness about intellectual disabilities, and challenges viewers: "Will you allow your conscience to ignore what you have just seen and heard or will you do something about it? It's up to you. The Department of Health and the government can do nothing without your support and encouragement." The final shot is of the children in the church service, earnestly reciting the Lord's Prayer.

The film is close to sixty years old, and it's easy to make fun of its heavy-handed message, preachy tone, and awkwardly staged scenes. It would be a mistake, though, to dismiss the power of its message. Scene after scene showed parents like mine that the hospital school was a clean,

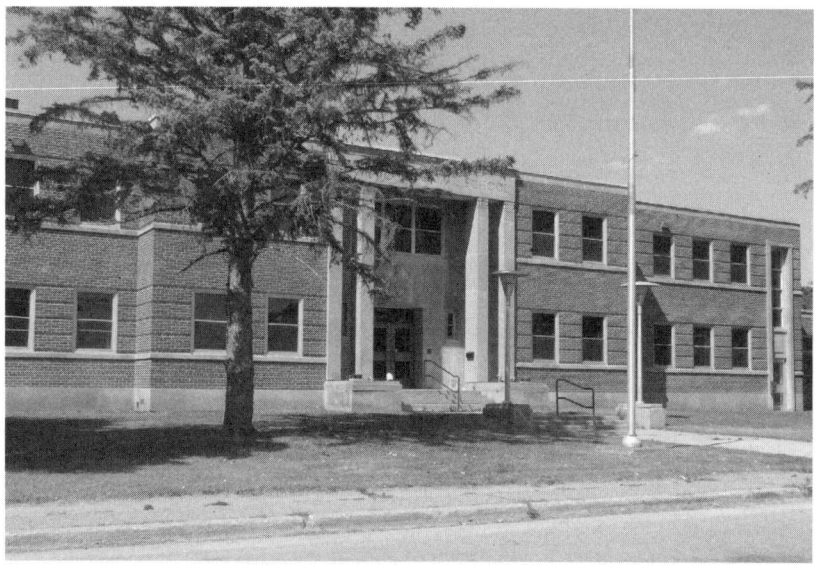

Though the facility is now in private hands, the main entrance to the hospital
school at Smiths Falls looks the same today as it did when Bill moved in.

kind, and safe place, where "afflicted people" could learn and develop as
far as possible, free of the pressures or constraints of the outside world,
and where children could have the opportunities denied to them in the
outer world — going to school, joining the Cub Scouts, learning music.
The experts knew how to take care of these children's needs better than
their own families; the watchwords for their care were *progress* and
happiness. What more could a parent want?

But I couldn't help but wonder what this film did *not* show. *Danny
and Nicky*, a National Film Board documentary produced in 1969, eight
years later, provides some of my answers.[11]

Fifty-five minutes long and directed by the Oscar-nominated docu-
mentarian Douglas Jackson, the film appeared at a time when activist
parents had made strides in keeping their children at home and in community day schools, rather than sending them to the institutions. The
documentary cuts back and forth between the lives of two boys with
Down syndrome: nine-year-old Danny, who lives at home and goes to a

new day school for children with intellectual disabilities; and fourteen-year-old Nicky, who lives at the Ontario Hospital School in Orillia. My brother Bill was thirteen the year the film came out, almost the same age as Nicky.

Nicky's story begins on the morning he moves from the children's ward, where he has lived for close to a decade, to the men's cottage. The children's ward is crowded, dingy, and sparsely equipped. The paint on the wall is patchy, the huge metal ward door is scraped and scarred, and very few toys are visible. Almost all the boys are wearing the same style of yellow-striped shirts, most likely a bulk purchase or a donation. But, institutional though it may be, this is the closest place Nicky has had to a home. It's where he grew from toddler to teenager, and where he serves as the kindly older brother to the younger boys. As the film opens, a jolly woman in a nurse's uniform announces that Nicky is about to go and urges the boys to say goodbye to him. Some give him a hug. A few kiss him. Others pay no attention. The film's narrator says that, in his new home, Nicky will have his first regular contact with boys his own age.

The move takes almost no time at all. The jolly nurse walks to the new ward with him, carrying his personal effects in a plastic bag about the size of a pillowcase under her arm. Nicky carries a large blue stuffed elephant, his treasured toy, under his. Together, the toy and the bag are all he has in the world. The nurse hands Nicky and his papers over to the men running the new ward, kisses him awkwardly, and leaves.

The supervisor in charge of the ward takes Nicky into the day room, the institutional equivalent of the family room in a private home. It is utterly bare except for a TV on a stand at one end and a row of hard chairs and wooden benches pushed against the walls on three sides of the room. Close to fifty boys, most of them sitting on the floor, look up when Nicky arrives. Three or four male attendants are in the ward, sitting on the chairs. Unlike the staff in the children's ward, the attendants here don't wear uniforms. Instead, they wear sport jackets and ties. The supervisor introduces Nicky to the crowd of boys, and tells them, "Remember the day you come in here, and you were all scared? Well Nicky's like that, and he wants you boys to be good to him."

He leads Nicky to a chair, sits him down beside two attendants, and goes to put Nicky's clothes away. One of the men asks Nicky if he wants to "sit in with the boys" on the floor. Nicky shakes his head and says he wants to stay on the chair. The other attendant says he can do as he wishes, but asks him again if he'd like join the writhing mass of boys on the floor. Nicky, still holding his elephant, gets up and walks to the other side of the room to sit on a bench. He puts the toy on the seat beside him.

In the next scene, a ward attendant gives Nicky a tour of the washroom. The door is badly banged up. Seven toilets sit in a row out in the open, with no privacy screens of any sort, and no toilet seats either. The attendant tells Nicky he can use any one he wishes. The washroom has a line of four or five sinks, one bathtub, and a row of showerheads hanging from an overhead pipe. Nicky looks nervous as he takes in his new bathroom.

Back in the day room, several boys are curious about Nicky's toy elephant, patting it and reaching for it. An attendant comes up to Nicky and asks if he can have it, explaining that the other boys will want to play with it, and that he will lock it in the office to keep it safe. Nicky says yes. The man takes it away. That's the last we see of Nicky's special toy.

The film cuts back and forth between Danny and Nicky's lives, showing where they sleep, where they go to school, how they spend their down time, where they eat their meals, et cetera. Danny's life looks remarkably ordinary. He goes to school and to the community pool, he has a hot dog with his mother at the mall, he feeds the squirrels with his father in the park, he eats dinner with the family, he plays with his brothers and sisters, he cuddles with his mother as the family watches television.

Nicky's days are spent entirely in the institution, and the scenes in the day room at Orillia are compelling. It's noisy and chaotic: lots of yelling, shoving, and nearly constant wrestling that starts off good-naturedly but sometimes gets out of hand. A few boys rock back and forth compulsively, shunning human contact. In one shot Nicky, still sitting on a bench, is crying. A boy puts his arm across his shoulders in a rough effort to comfort him. Another boy, his shirt torn, is also crying, hurt in all the roughhousing. Suddenly, a boy rushes up to Nicky and yanks him off the bench. Nicky, who clearly does not want to wrestle, ducks him and sits down. The boy comes after him again. Nicky looks confused, overwhelmed, and scared.

At one point an attendant tells all the boys to move to the benches so that the floor is empty. He is holding a box of candy and smiling. Nicky looks confused, but the other boys seem to know what's coming: the man will throw the candies in the air and the kids will scramble for them. When the man tosses the candy, the other boys clamber after the pieces, jumping and bumping and grabbing and pushing and shouting. The fastest and the strongest get to the candy first; the smaller, or slower, or less aggressive boys are shoved aside. Nicky looks terrified. He stays on the bench with another boy and timidly holds out his hand. No candy comes his way. He stands up and holds his hand out a bit more boldly. Again, nothing comes his way. At the end of the scramble, the attendant asks if anyone did not get any candy. Several boys shoot their hands up in the air, far more quickly than Nicky. "Don't push," the attendant tells the boys, "everyone will get some." Nicky, back on the bench, smacks his knees in frustration.

Throughout the film, the attendants continue to press Nicky to sit on the floor with the other boys. The message is clear: Nicky must not hold himself apart, or see himself as anything other than just another boy on the ward. If he won't scramble on the floor for candy, he won't get candy. The only way to get by is to be like everyone else. Nicky holds out for a while. But eventually, inevitably, he gives in and moves to the floor.

In the scenes filmed in his classroom, Nicky seems happier and more engaged than in the day room. The lesson of the day is "can" and "cannot," and the teacher asks a girl to tell her something she can do. The girl says, "I can sing." Asked to name something she cannot do, the girl says she cannot turn herself into a blackboard. The teacher agrees, and asks her to read a sentence on the board and decide whether it is "can" or "cannot." She does, and she gets it right. The teacher then asks Nicky to read a sentence: "Nicky can run and jump." He stumbles over the words, but with a bit of prompting he correctly identifies it as a "can." He smiles. He also works on his writing, copying his name neatly three times per line in his notebook.

Back in the day room, two chatty brothers — they look like twins, with oversized glasses, big ears, and buck-toothed grins — befriend Nicky and fill him in on the way things work in the ward. They tell him not to take the fights seriously. It's mostly play fighting, they say, but if things get out of hand, Nicky should go find an attendant. "When people hit you, Nicky, go and tell the staff, okay? And the staff will cut them down to size," one of the brothers says. They also tell him to pay no attention to "smart boys" who say threatening things like "Do you want to die young?" And they warn Nicky that if he misbehaves, the staff will "give you a little tap." The brothers then ask him about his family, whether he has any pets, and what they eat. One asks, "What's the mostest thing and important thing that you like the best and that's safe for you?" Nicky replies with a shy smile, "Mommy." Later, these brothers and a few other boys entertain the rest by singing a popular children's song. Nicky, by now sitting on the floor with the others, listens. Afterward, some boys turn somersaults, while others sing. Nicky stands on his head.

At the end of the day, the attendants call out each boy by name and give him his toothbrush. The boys brush their teeth in groups of two or three per sink. It's fast and messy work, with spit flying everywhere. The attendant hurries them along so the next group can use the sinks. Showers are also a group activity, with boys bumping and shouting and sliding and playing on the tiles.

At eight-thirty p.m., it's time for bed. The TV goes off and the boys walk from the day room into the bedroom. It has long rows of beds — no chairs or other furniture — and the hospital-green walls badly need a coat of paint. The boys sit on the side of their beds and change into pajamas.

An attendant yells at them to fold their clothes. That done, Nicky climbs into his bed. The attendant turns out the light and exits through the day room, which is a mess, covered in scraps of paper and random bits of trash. No one says goodnight.

Nicky looks exhausted at the end of his first day on the new ward. No one has been deliberately cruel to him, though the wrestling has been pretty violent at times. The attendants are mostly passive, except during the candy scramble. Their job seems to consist of sticking to the timetable and preventing rough play from getting out of hand. Otherwise, they don't talk to the boys. Some of the boys on the ward are genuinely friendly, others are less so, and a few are aggressive. But what stays with me, watching the film, is the noise—the unrelenting howl of fifty young teenage boys with too much time on their hands and too little to occupy it. Nicky has not had a moment for reflection or respite from the crowd. The boys strip down to shower in groups, put on their pajamas in groups, eat in groups, brush their teeth in groups, and spend every moment in each other's company. Every scene is deafening. Nicky has no choice but to go along. His only choice, it seems, is which open toilet to use.

When Danny goes to bed, his mother tucks him in and gives him a kiss. When Nicky goes to bed, he is alone in a crowd of children. It's hard to find any signs of the "progress and happiness" promised in *One on Every Street* in Nicky's constrained and narrow life.

The renowned sociologist Erving Goffman applied the term *total institution* to places where people work, sleep, and play in a singularly enclosed and regulated life, conforming to rules and patterns of behaviour designed to fulfill the official aims of the institution.[12] When someone enters a total institution, Goffman writes, every aspect of pre-institutional life is erased and replaced with the routines and demands of life in the institution. He calls this process "mortification of the self." Mortification of the self, he explains, attacks identity. It strips away possessions, comforts, communication channels to the world outside, and the power to make decisions. The newcomer must learn how to conform, and how to win rewards and avoid punishments. Watching newcomers go through the process reinforces the status quo for those who have gone through it themselves.

Nicky's move to a new ward in *Danny and Nicky* is a portrait of mortification of the self in action.

Some inmates of a total institution withdraw, Goffman writes, while others rebel and some simply embrace the rules. It's easy to see all three responses in the boys in Nicky's ward. No matter how they adapt, though, institutional life exacts a price. And Nicky and the other boys paid it.

My brother did, too.

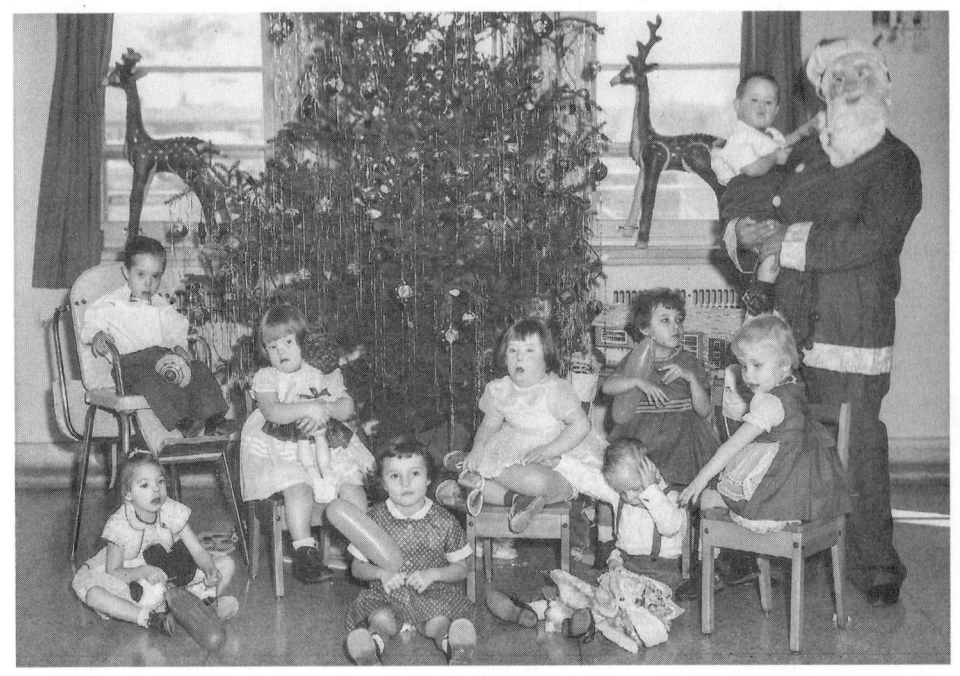

The institution asked my parents for permission to use this photograph
of Bill — he's in Santa's arms — and other children as its 1959 Christmas card.
"This is certainly a very charming group and I am sure you will enjoy
keeping the photograph," the superintendent wrote.

Chapter 5

"LITTLE, WELL NOURISHED **MONGOLIAN**"

I have no memories of Mom and Dad taking Billy away; nor do my brother or sister. How do you prepare your toddler to leave his home and family? How do you prepare your other children to say goodbye to their baby brother? How do you prepare yourself? Mary, who at nine was the one most likely to remember his departure, says, "I suspect that Mom and Dad did it without telling us beforehand. I don't even remember them explaining where Billy was, although they must have."

The crib disappeared from Bill's room and went straight into the trash. Mom said the finish was too corroded by vomit for it to be passed on to anyone. After years of living in various configurations of shared rooms, Mary, Bob, and I were shuffled again. This time, we each got a bedroom of our own. Mary was in what had been the maid's room, I was in the middle room that had for a time been Bill's, and Bob was in the big double room at the end of the hall. Our cousin David remembers once asking Bob why his bedroom had two beds. Bob replied that one was his and the other was for his brother, as if expecting him to come home at any moment.

Mom had always known, whether she admitted it or not, that she and Dad would send Billy to Smiths Falls one day. And, once she filled out the forms in November of 1958, she knew that day was approaching quickly. But knowing it would happen *someday* is a far different thing from having it happen *today*. In a flash on a cold, late-winter day, he was gone. The silence in the house must have been deafening. I don't think

I ever asked her directly what she remembered of the day she and Dad took Billy away, or how the rest of us reacted to his sudden disappearance. That was deliberate on my part. Asking her about it would have been like picking at a poorly healed scar — though whether it was her scar I was protecting or my own, I can't say for certain.

With Billy gone, she had her life back. No more worrying about him vomiting on the barber or in the car or at the grocery store or on us; no more keeping a brave face as strangers averted their eyes or clucked over the poor afflicted child; no more trouble finding babysitters or once-a-week house cleaners or someone to watch him while she went to the hairdresser. She had three "normal" kids now, just like the other mothers in our neighbourhood. She and Dad were free to resume "normal" life, a happy mix of work, family time, and socializing.

Of course, removing your toddler from your home doesn't erase him from your heart. Mom's freedom came at a heavy cost: crushing, relentless guilt. It tweaked her conscience whenever she saw a family that had kept their child with Down syndrome at home. It drove her to tears one September when she forgot to send money to the institution for his birthday party. It morphed into anxiety when I was pregnant with my own children. It haunted her dreams. While Dad asserted that sending Bill to Smiths Falls was the right choice, in those early months of 1959, Mom was in turmoil. She was mourning the child she felt she had abandoned, yet relieved to be rid of the burden of caring for him. She was happy to have more time for her other children, yet missing her baby. She was feeling terrible about feeling either relieved or happy, and struggling to come to terms with it all with no outside support.

An additional cruelty came from the institution: we were to have no contact with Billy for at least a month. This was, Mom says, to give him time to adjust. But it also was a message: Billy was the institution's child now, not ours. Mom never forgot the pain this supposedly well-intentioned ban caused. "I cannot describe how awful we felt," she wrote in a letter to the three of us more than twenty-five years later.

It must have been a long, strange month for us all.

When Billy disappeared from our home, we disappeared from each other's daily lives. We had almost no idea of how he spent his days, what he ate, where he slept, what made him happy or sad or scared. I hoped that his resident file would help fill in the gaps. Records record things the institution or individual making the record considers worth recording. In other words, they're a judgment from the record maker on what matters and what doesn't. Bill's record, especially in his early years, is long on empirical data and short on anything else. This is in line with the medical model of institutional care; if the institution's job is to provide treatment to people with a medical condition, the condition and the treatment take centre stage. The fears or hopes or feelings of the person who has the condition are of far less interest.

Bill's ward admission record describes him as "clean, well nourished and no vermin." His teeth — ten upper and ten lower — were good. His clothing was clean. He had an umbilical hernia. His parents were "co-operative." He was 31.5 inches tall and weighed twenty-five pounds, both below average for a child his age. The doctor who signed the form described Bill's general health as "good." Nonetheless, he started him on a ten-day course of the antibiotic Gantrisin, perhaps to prevent possible infections. Five days later, the same doctor gave him a more thorough physical exam, including Bill's head measurements — circumference 45.1 cm, length 15 cm, width 12 cm. The doctor noted that both testicles were descended, but the left one was atrophied. His summary of my brother's condition: "Little, well nourished Mongolian."

In addition to cataloguing his physical condition, Bill's admission record tallies his possessions. A form carefully filled out by a clerk says he came with one snowsuit, one helmet-style hat, one cardigan sweater, five sets of overalls, one pair of short pants, six T-shirts, three sleepers, four undershirts, five bibs, seven pairs of socks, two pairs of boots, and three pairs of plastic pants. That's it. No toys, and nothing personal.

But his file offers almost no answers for how Bill reacted to the move. The change in his life must have been incomprehensible. Everyone and everything he knew and loved was gone. His home, his parents, his sisters, and his brother had disappeared, and he was in a strange new place with strange new people. His "clinical record" for 1959—the form that details life on ward—contains brief notes from staff, some handwritten and some typed, summarizing his first few days in the institution. On February 18, the day he was admitted, he "eagerly" ate "veg and chicken, pears, cookie and milk." On February 19, 20, and 21, he had no temperature, ate well, moved his bowels, seemed happy, and played around the ward. The handwritten note for February 22 says he was "very rough this a.m." and "pulled another small patient over in his chair, thereby acquiring a bump on forehead." (The typed version makes clear it was the other child who "acquired" the bump, not Bill.) As a result, "Billy kept in playpen." On February 23, he had a quiet day. "Takes any foods he likes very well. Will spit out food he dislikes. Enjoys getting into things. Throws toys around. Bad tempered at times." On February 24, "behaviour much the same. A quiet day. Grinds his teeth often. Set in his ways." On February 25, "plays well in playpen. He plays rough." The word *rough* was not one any of us in the family had ever applied to Bill. He was undersized and physically timid. The rough behaviour was probably a sign of emotional turmoil—he must have been feeling more and more desperate as each day passed, lost and angry and confused about why it was taking so long for Mom and Dad to come and get him. But that's just a guess; the people taking care of him made no further comments on his emotional state.

In fact, there are no further entries at all until June 1, when the clinical record reports he was in isolation on his ward for dysentery.

—

According to a handwritten visitor log in his file, no one went to see Billy until April 18, two months to the day after our parents admitted him. A second visit took place the following day, April 19, and a third on April 23. These dates are confusing; if they are accurate, either Mom waited a full month longer than required before visiting or the ban on family visits lasted a month longer than she recalled. It's also hard to understand why she would make three visits in less than a week. Perhaps our parents wanted to see Billy by themselves before bringing the rest of us along. Perhaps they had appointments with someone from the team in charge of his care. Or perhaps the clerk recording the dates made a mistake, and the first visit was on March 18, not April 18.

April 19 was a Saturday that year, and that was probably the first time the whole family went to see Bill. My memories of those family visits pile into each other and are impossible to untangle, but in the early years, they followed the same pattern. One Saturday a month, we climbed into Dad's car and headed west out along Carling Avenue, then south on Highway 15. We passed farms and swamps and woodlots, the stone church in Franktown that looked to us like a castle, and, about an hour after leaving the house, we got to the northern edge of Smiths Falls. It was, and still is, a hardscrabble town. Smiths Falls began as cluster of buildings around a sawmill, and grew into a village in the late 1820s when the Rideau Canal was being built. The Canadian Pacific Railway, a farm implements maker, and a foundry were the major employers in the twentieth century, but the Depression and Second World War hit them all hard. Grimy storefronts, budget shops, garages, and coffee shops lined Beckwith, the main street. We would get to know it well. To get to Bill's, however, we turned left before getting to the centre of town. We drove alongside the Rideau River for a while, passed under the railway bridge, turned left onto the institution grounds, headed up the long, tree-lined drive to the main building, parked, and went inside.

The institution was huge, low, and brown. Architects describe it as built in a "severely handsome Art Deco" style,[1] though I never saw much handsome about it. Square grey pillars flanked the door to the main building, but otherwise it had that stripped-down, low-profile, brown-brick look of Ontario's post-war institutional architecture.

Mary, Bob, and I knew Billy lived in something called a ward with other children his age, but we never saw it when we were children, so we had no idea what a ward at Smiths Falls looked like. This too was institution policy: families were not allowed into the wards. When we

wanted to visit Billy, Mom had to phone a few days ahead to let the staff
know we were coming. We checked in at the front desk and were sent to a
dimly lit visitors' lounge that pouched out to one side of the long, central
corridor. The stale air smelled strongly of disinfectant, with undertones
of cafeteria food, diapers, and body odour. We waited while someone
went to get Billy.

Those waits were always nerve-wracking. Though I tried not to stare,
I found it hard not to. I knew hospitals because Dad worked in one and
I had gone there with him several times. I knew schools because I went
to one. But this hospital school looked like neither. I also knew this was
a home for children, but none of the homes I knew looked or smelled
this way. And some of the so-called children were as big as adults. A few
looked as old as Nana.

The hospital school was crowded, with a constant flow of people up
and down the corridor past the visitors' lounge. The residents—officially
known as patients, though everyone seemed to call them kids—had every
kind of intellectual disability, from mild to severe, and a fair number had
physical disabilities too. Those with Down syndrome looked familiar, in
that they looked like Billy, but the others were variations on the human
form I had never seen before. There were kids whose heads were too big
and kids whose heads were too small; kids who needed wheelchairs or
crutches or gurneys or other contraptions to get around; kids who moved
in jerks and bounced off the wall as they walked; kids who lumbered in
a straight, fast line down the hall; kids whose faces looked incomplete or
distorted or not quite set properly; kids who were utterly silent and didn't
move; kids who yelled or laughed or cried for no reason I could see. The
ones I found most fascinating, though, were the ones who looked, as far
as I could tell, pretty ordinary. While waiting for Bill, I played a secret
game of "guess the patient," trying to figure out who lived there and
who was simply visiting. I never told anyone about this game, because I
knew it was rude to stare. But I had trouble understanding how our Billy
fit into this place, and the game was an attempt to figure it out. This

hospital school was another world from any I had imagined. It was odd. It was surprising. It was scary, a bit. It was fascinating.

Eventually — and it was usually just five minutes or so — we'd hear Billy's short, rapid footsteps pattering down the hall. He'd come around the corner and run straight into Mom's arms, smiling and crowing with delight. Hugs to Dad followed, then to rest of us. Billy was always clean and wearing good clothes when he came down for a visit, probably dressed up by the staff for the occasion. The girls in the visitors' lounge seeing their own families were dressed up, too, in fancy frocks. Invariably in those early visits, Billy threw up a bit — as the doctors predicted, he eventually outgrew the problem — and Mom always had tissues at the ready.

It's still chilly in Smiths Falls in April, so we probably spent that first visit in the visitors' lounge. Later, on nicer days, we drove to Victoria Park, beside the Rideau Canal off Lombard Street in the centre of town. It had a playground, boat docks, picnic tables, a creek where Bob and I searched for crayfish, and a yellow, two-seater airplane on a pillar. (I learned later that the plane was a Second World War–era Harvard Trainer.) We sat at a picnic table and ate the sandwiches Mom packed, then Mary, Bob, and I ran off to play on the swings. Billy stayed with Mom and Dad, eating green grapes one by one, and smiling and nodding and enjoying being with them. In the winter, or on rainy days, or if Billy had a cold, we had our picnic in the lounge. Those visits tended to be shorter; the lounge was often crowded and noisy, and there was nothing for Mary, Bob, and me to do. Park visits were better.

We often took Billy to Beckwith Street to shop for new shoes or other things he needed. When a Burger King opened at the north end of Beckwith Street some years later, it became Bill's favourite restaurant. Bill's vocabulary was very limited, but *hamburger*, *french fries*, and *Coke* were words he said with gusto. Another favourite spot was the Hershey chocolate factory, which opened in the 1960s and became the town's second largest employer, after the hospital school. Bill liked candy, but he didn't like it when the chocolate dripped or got onto his hands or clothing. He liked peanut butter cups, probably because they came in their own little paper containers.

Bill, who grew from sturdy toddler to chubby child to stocky teenager, ate fastidiously when he was out with us. At home in the institution, I learned from his file, his table manners were much less polished. He insisted on licking his dishes, cups, and cutlery during and after a meal. But when he was out with us, his manners were impeccable. Unwrapping his drinking straw was a ritual. He carefully squeezed ketchup packets onto his burger wrapper. He ate his french fries with a fork, one at a time, dipping each into the ketchup. His only lapse was licking up the leftover ketchup when the fries were finished.

We usually took Billy back to the institution in the middle of the afternoon. Again, we didn't go to his ward—someone collected him at the same visitors' lounge where we picked him up in the morning—and then we headed home, back down the long driveway, right onto Queen Street, north on Highway 15, then east into Ottawa.

The drive home was usually very quiet. Visiting days often ended with Mom retreating to her bedroom early and shutting the door.

The monthly family visits continued for years. But, one by one, members of the family began to skip the occasional visit. When we were in high school, Mary or I would go every other time, or we'd go as long as we didn't have something else going on that day, or just at holidays, or just for one of the institution's periodic family days. After we left home for university, we saw Bill rarely. Dad's visits dropped off as well, down to a couple of times a year. Bob was Mom's regular companion until he headed to university; after that, he rarely went. Mom, however, visited Bill faithfully, month after month after month. The visitor log in Bill's file shows that, between April 1959 and June 1967, she visited 121 times. The log ends there; the visits did not.

Many visits were pleasant; others less so. Sometimes Billy was cranky, and sometimes we were bored. Occasionally Billy had impressively loud temper tantrums, usually when Mom wanted him to do something he

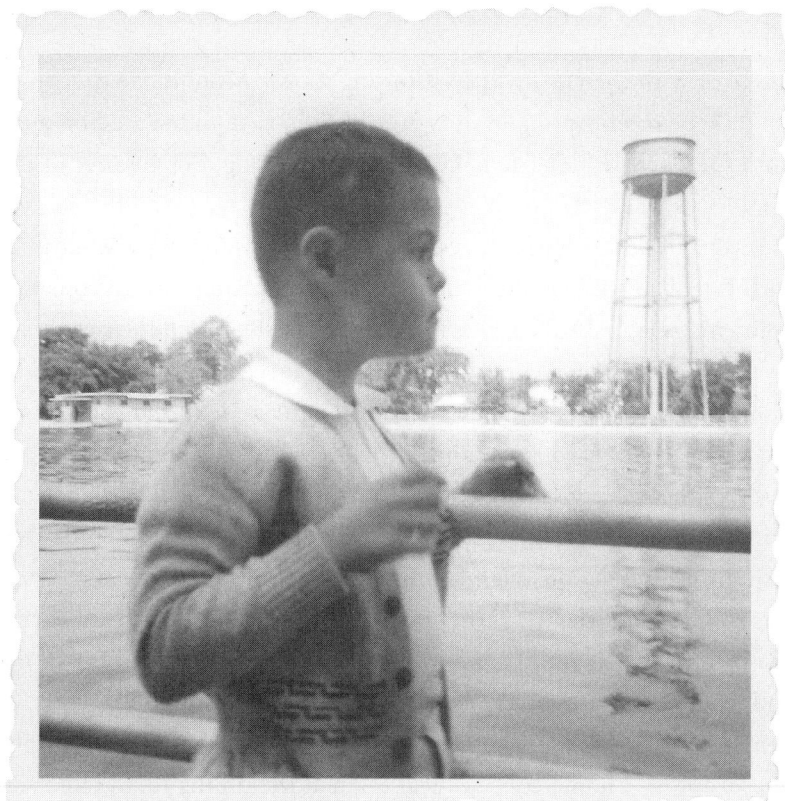

Almost all the photographs we have of our visits with Bill were
taken at the same spot, Victoria Park beside the Rideau Canal.
What makes this one unusual is that I was the photographer,
taking this snapshot with my first camera.

didn't want to do, like try on a new sweater or put away the grapes before
they were all gone. Bob recalls one visit when Bill was a teenager that
ended with Mom crying all the way home. But after the first visit, Mom
wrote to us later, she was relieved. Billy was "happy and well cared for" at
the hospital school; he seemed to have adjusted to life outside our family.
And we were beginning to adjust to our family without Bill.

—

Alone or with the family, the visitor log shows, Mom made six trips to see Billy between April and mid-June of 1959, then didn't see him again until October 1. I don't remember a gap that long, but I do recall that summer. It was a hard one.

Every marriage has its stresses, and the decision about what to do with Billy had strained our parents' relationship almost to the breaking point. Years later, Dad confided it was the worst crisis in their marriage.

Our parents were a good couple. They loved each other but, more importantly, they liked each other's company and trusted each other's judgment. (Except when it came to politics — Mom leaned Liberal and Dad, a life-long Conservative, considered John Diefenbaker the greatest prime minister of all time.) As a couple and as parents, they took their responsibilities seriously and supported each other's decisions. Mom was in charge of the kids, the menu, and the household. Dad earned the income and made the big-money decisions, like which car to buy and where to go on vacation. He worked long hours and his work was demanding. She made sure he came home to a clean and comfortable house, and to a home-cooked meal eaten at the dining room table with children whose hair was combed and whose homework was done. Their life was not simply a matter of comfortable routines, however: each lit up when the other came into the room. They always greeted each other with a kiss. They rarely argued.

When it came to Billy, though, they disagreed at an absolutely fundamental level. Mom saw him as her baby, as much a part of her family as the rest of us, despite his disability; Dad saw him as a cruel mistake that threatened to be a drain on us all. In the end, Dad's wishes to send him away from the rest of us prevailed, but neither of them believed they had "won" when they took Billy to Smiths Falls. The fact is, there was no winning on this issue: merely the hope that Dad's choice would turn out to be a wise one for everyone. It must have been agonizing for them.

In June of 1959, just a few months after sending Billy away, Mom and Dad sailed to Europe for a six-week vacation. This was a chance to escape the demands of family, enjoy uninterrupted time together, and, though they never put it quite that bluntly, repair their marriage.

Our house, which had been so full just a few months earlier, suddenly felt empty. Nana came to stay with us, but she was no substitute for our parents. She didn't drive, she was partly deaf and therefore hard to talk to, and she was a dreadful cook. School was out, so the routines that gave structure to our lives were gone. Our world shrank in on itself. Bob, the youngest and most sensitive of us, took it the hardest. Mary and I were old enough, I think, to understand that Mom and Dad would come back, even if Billy would not. I'm not sure Bob, who turned five a week or two after they left, had the same confidence. A birthday without your parents there just seemed wrong. My birthday was three weeks after Bob's, and the best gift for me was knowing they would be home soon.

Abandonment runs in more than one direction. Mom tore herself up over abandoning Bill, but she and Dad apparently were oblivious to the possibility that the rest of us might feel abandoned when they disappeared from our lives that summer. Mary, Bob, and I had lost half our family that year — temporarily, in the case of our parents, but for long enough to feel that our family was somehow broken. Perhaps our parents knew this, perhaps not. Or perhaps they felt that, unless they took some time to repair their own relationship, the family might break apart in another way.

Mom and Dad returned from Europe full of smiles and with armloads of presents: watches, Swiss army knives, a fancy toy fire truck, dolls in colourful traditional costumes. But nothing gave us more joy than the relief of having our family together again.

Or at least, mostly together.

After our parents took Billy to Smiths Falls, my brother never came home again. Never. As children, Mary, Bob, and I accepted this. I think we believed it was against the rules for him to visit us. Not so, I learned later. There were no rules against bringing him home for a visit. We could easily have taken him home for a meal, a day, a weekend, or a holiday. We could have taken him to the cottage to play in the shallows of the Ottawa River, or to enjoy burgers and hot dogs on the deck.

Some families dropped their children off at the institution and simply left them there. Former Rideau Regional resident David McKillop, who was admitted at the age of four and a half, didn't see his parents again until he was sixteen.[2] Some families, like ours, visited but didn't bring their children home. Others brought their children home for weekends or holidays or vacations. In fact, by the mid-1970s, the institution was actively encouraging visits home. My parents received a form letter at one point announcing a new mini-bus service to Ottawa from the institution. It proposed three specific weekends for home visits — one in May, one in June, and one in July — and asked whether our family would like to take advantage of the offer. Mom ticked the box saying "No, I am not interested in having my child participate in this program," and sent the form back. The woman who was Bill's primary counsellor around 1990-91 lived in Ottawa and offered, more than once, to drive him to the city with her and drop him off at my parents' home. They never took her up on the offer.

It's not that they never talked about bringing Bill home to visit — though I don't think they ever talked about it with Mary, Bob, or me. The idea "came up again and again," Mom confided in her 1985 letter to us. "Your father always said, 'No.'" Dad had a never-ending set of reasons why. The one he trotted out most often was that the Rideau Regional Centre was Bill's home, and bringing him to our home in Ottawa would only confuse him. Dad applied that argument to birthdays, Christmases, and any other holiday. But there was more. "First we didn't want to confuse him, then it wasn't safe with electric appliances, plumbing and locks," Mom wrote. "Remember, Bill was agile and manually efficient — he thought it fun to knock lamps over and pull out plugs." The waterfront ruled out visits to the family cottage on the Ottawa River: "He loved the water and I don't know how we would manage him at the cottage if he decided to swim — he is very strong and not always easy to control."

Mom knew that these were excuses, and pretty lame ones at that. But Dad was adamant. He had worked very hard to convince everyone that sending Bill away was the right thing to so, and had prevailed only when the family was in crisis. I think he was terrified that if Bill had a good visit at home, Mom — or perhaps one or more of the rest of us — would want to keep him there: first for a weekend, then for a vacation, and after that who knows? He wanted to avoid that possibility at all costs. "In his practice he had seen families under great stress because the retarded child needed and got the major share of the mother's attention," Mom later observed. Coming from an ear, nose, and throat doctor, this was an odd observation, but he was probably looking for evidence wherever he could find it, including among his patients and colleagues. Mom decided not to make the issue a deal breaker. "Lest I give the impression your father was the villain of the piece, I confess I didn't argue too hard for my views," she noted.

In the winter of 1973-74, Mom had a heart attack that landed her in the hospital for weeks, and left her with permanent damage. Any serious talk of bringing Bill home stopped. But, years later, she wrote, "My main regret is that we didn't bring him home for visits and so keep him a part of the family."

Bill did make it to Ottawa for the occasional weekend family visit in the early 1990s, but not with us. His primary counsellor, Sandy Baker Lennox, told me she sometimes took him home to stay with her and her family. He also went to her pre-wedding stag party — "best party ever," she said, with Bill dancing almost non-stop — and to her wedding. "Oh, I loved him," she said. "He was part of my family."[3]

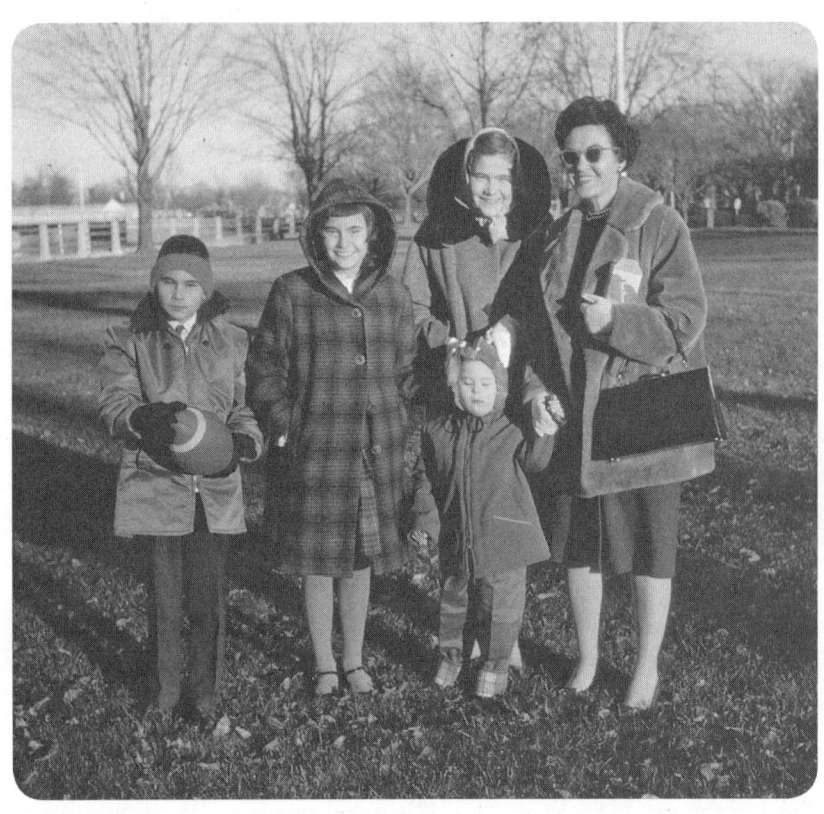

By 1962, the year my father snapped this family photo, other parents
were beginning to question the institutional approach. My parents,
however, accepted the idea that the Ontario Hospital School gave
Bill his best chance for "progress and happiness."

Chapter 6
"VERY **INSTITUTIONALIZED**"

The government promised that the Ontario hospital schools would give children like Bill their best chance for "progress and happiness." My parents liked that idea, though they had no idea what kind of "progress" their toddler son would likely make. The experts at the hospital school, they hoped, would tell them what to expect.

In May of 1959, the institution's psychological experts set out to assess the extent of Billy's intellectual impairment. Using IQ and social development tests, observation, and an extensive family history, the hospital school wanted to judge what he was capable of learning or doing—a judgment that would help determine the kind of care he'd receive. The experts and specialists met in June of that year to go over the results. According to a report on that meeting, included in his resident file, his IQ was 38 and his mental age was that of a one-year-old.

"He is a cheerful and happy little lad who gets along very well with the other children," the report said. "He walks about without help. He obeys simple commands and is able to say a few words. His toilet habits are not established and he is starting now to feed himself. He is functioning at the lower end of the imbecile range of intelligence." The term *imbecile* hit me like a smack to the side of the head. I had braced myself for the disparaging language I knew I'd find in the material from the nineteenth and early twentieth century, but to see it in an expert report from the late 1950s was a surprise. I later learned that, at the time of Bill's first assessment, it was a category of "mental deficiency" that had been in use for decades. People with IQs between 90 and 70 were considered dull or borderline, and anyone whose IQ was below that was classified as feeble-minded. There were three types of feeble-minded people: morons (IQs of 50–69), imbeciles (IQs of 20–49), and idiots (IQs below 20).[1] Terms like these convey not just an assessment of an intellectual impairment, but a judgment about the individual who has the impairment. It's shocking to see those words used so casually by people whose jobs were, ostensibly, to help Bill reach the best of his abilities, but they fit the tenor of the times.

The report recommended institutional and nursing care for Bill, "habit training" (how to dress himself, use the toilet, etc.), and "ward school attendance." Children with higher IQs went to on-site classrooms for their education. Ward school was for the rest. The superintendent of the Ontario Hospital School at Orillia came up with the curriculum for ward schooling in the 1930s, featuring play therapy, music, calisthenics, and "industrial classes."[2] There are no ward school records in Bill's file, unfortunately, though it seems likely from other reports that Bill's "industrial" lessons were how to use a floor mop.

A little over three years later, when Billy was six, the experts assessed him again. This time his IQ was 23 and his mental age was one year, five months. The psychologist who tested him reported that his language skills were extremely limited—"could not speak other than to attempt to say 'mama' and 'dada'"—and his comprehension was poor for someone of his mental age. "He did not understand verbal instructions, questions or the use of common objects. His attention span was very short both for test problems and for his play activities, which seemed aimless. He showed no immediate or past memory." The report concluded that Billy was "functioning in the idiot range of intelligence."

IQ and mental age tests are far from perfect instruments for measuring intelligence, especially when assessing young, mainly non-verbal children who have spent the bulk of their life in an institution. But this report indicates that Bill not only had *not* progressed at Smiths Falls, but had regressed. His IQ had slid fifteen points. His language skills had eroded.

His attention and memory skills had declined, too. Three years in the hospital school, and he was more impaired than ever.

Bill never took another IQ test. His next assessment, in 1976, said no formal testing was possible: "An attempt was made to get him to complete items on the WAIS (Wechsler Adult Intelligence Scale) but with little success." In 1982, his IQ was estimated at "less than 30."

So much for progress. What about the happiness part of the equation? The 1962 assessment offers a single comment: "The ward staff reported that he was well socialized and happy on the ward."

Clinical reports on Bill in the 1960s — a few brief lines at most, and compiled infrequently by a range of staff members on his ward — appear to equate happiness with good behaviour. Report after report noted that Bill was generally cheerful, generally obedient, and generally followed simple instructions. He learned how to use the toilet and to dress himself. He liked to watch TV, play catch, chew gum, go for walks. He liked ward school, though the reports suggest he learned very little. He got along with other children on the ward, though he made no close friends and he tended to tease the others. He sought approval and affection from the staff.

He was also, the reports say, "stubborn." This word shows up in his file early and often over the years, and it seems to have had a particular meaning. Bill had a very strong sense of order. He clung to routine. He hated change. He resisted, often loudly, any deviation from how he thought the events of a day should unfold. If someone tried to get him to do something that offended his sense of order, Bill objected. He roared, pouted, stomped his feet, or slid to a heap on the floor. If he was made to comply anyway, he fussed and groaned and moved as slowly as possible.

Nobody seemed particularly interested in figuring out why he was so resistant to change. What mattered, the notes in his file suggest, was whether he obeyed the rules, followed the routines, and didn't cause too much trouble for the staff. If he did all that, and especially if he did it with a smile, the staff concluded he was happy.

The notes about Bill's life on the wards during his childhood years are frustratingly skimpy. His medical file is far more extensive, but just as frustrating. That's because it records a treatment but not necessarily the reason for the treatment. Packed with residents, the hospital school was a breeding ground for contagious diseases. In his first year there, his medical file shows, the doctors put Bill on antibiotics at least eleven times. But, aside from a recorded case of bronchitis in April 1959, there's no indication of what they were treating. Bill came down with measles in 1961. He had a couple of respiratory infections. Hepatitis A, a contagious viral liver disease spread by eating or drinking food or water contaminated with infected feces, ran rampant through all the hospital schools in the late 1950s and early 1960s. A single 1981 test result in Bill's medical file reported that he had hepatitis A antibodies, suggesting he'd had the disease at some point, but I found nothing to indicate when. He had countless staphylococcus bacterial infections, which usually showed up as styes in his eyes and boils on his buttocks, breast, and armpits, and once as cellulitis, a serious infection of the skin and the soft tissue beneath it. At one point, he was diagnosed with chicken pox. That made no sense, as he'd already had the disease when he was living at home with us. Most probably what they recorded as chicken pox was a bad outbreak of boils instead.

Chillingly, a note in his medical file in 1961 says Bill "may have restraint jacket p.r.n.," which means when the staff decides it's necessary. It's hard to imagine the circumstances under which a timid and undersized five-year-old would need restraints, and there's no record of anyone using them on Bill. But it's also hard to imagine prescribing restraints unless someone planned to use them, and the casualness of the order makes me shudder.

Institutional life was rough, especially after Bill moved out of the infants and toddlers ward in late 1962 or early 1963 and into one of the large, crowded, barracks-like wards typical of the hospital school system. We saw signs of this on just about every visit. "It was very painful to see the bruises and scratches on his face from the other children as he grew older," Mom recalled in her letter. Bill broke a finger one year and a collarbone the next. He needed stitches for a deep cut on his head a few months later. On family visits, we all noticed the deep gouges on Bill's face and arms, the kind you get from someone else's fingernail. He had lots of bruises too. Given the way he lived—in wards with too many children and too few supervisors; with boys who had behavioural problems as well as intellectual disabilities, and who had too much time on their hands and too little to occupy it; in the type of institution where making children scramble on the floor for candies was seen as a happy diversion, and where staff could punish misbehaviour physically—this was no surprise. The staff told my parents this was just normal wear and tear, and my parents believed them. By the time he was an adult, his skin was criss-crossed with scars.

Another problem, a curious one, began showing up when he was nine or ten—Bill was losing his hair. The loss began with his eyelashes, then spread to his eyebrows and his head. By 1966, he had so many bald patches that he was sent to the doctor. "The question is—is this hair just being pulled out by the boy himself which is usually the case, or is this ringworm of the scalp?" the medical consultant wrote. "There are no other cases reported on the ward where he has been staying for many months. Examination with a magnifying glass shows several fractured hairs which would suggest pulling out the hair by himself." At one point, the medical staff treated Bill for a fungal infection of the scalp; at another point for threadworm, an intestinal parasite that sometimes shows up on the scalp. Neither treatment seems to have made a difference. That made sense, in the end: Bill was losing his hair because he was twisting, rubbing, or pulling it out himself. A photo the institution took of him at twenty is startling: by this point he had the same thick, dark eyebrows as Bob and Dad, but the photo shows a dark eyebrow over his right eye and nothing over the left.

Psychologists call hair pulling an impulse control disorder. Some impulse control disorders are pretty benign, like biting your nails, while others can be dangerous, like compulsive shoplifting or setting fires. The cause of this kind of behaviour is unknown. According to the US-based non-profit known as Mental Health America, hair pulling shows up more often in girls than boys, and typically appears between the ages of nine and thirteen: "The onset of this disorder may be preceded or accompanied by various emotional states, such as feelings of anxiety or boredom." A stressful event such as abuse, family conflict, or death may trigger it.[3] The Mayo Clinic says that some people pull out their hair intentionally to relieve tension or distress, while others do it unconsciously, and some do both. The cause is unclear, but a combination of genetic and environmental factors is probably responsible.[4] People who have this disorder may have other conditions as well, such as depression, anxiety, or obsessive-compulsive disorder.

People with intellectual disabilities are not, of course, immune to mental health disorders. In fact, the US National Down Syndrome Society estimates that at least half of people with Down syndrome will face a significant mental health problem at some point during their life. Anxiety is a very common one, showing up in both children and adults. So is obsessive-compulsive or repetitive behaviour: "Increased level of restlessness and worry may lead the child or adult to behave in a very rigid manner, even resulting in a state of being 'stuck'.... They also engage in repetitive, compulsive, as well as ritualistic behaviors that raise the question of obsessive-compulsive disorder."[5] The term *stuck* refers to the idea that the individual needs to follow a specific routine or complete a particular action to prevent being overwhelmed by anxiety.

Beyond ruling out fungus or worms, no one at Smiths Falls seemed particularly interested in figuring out *why* Bill was pulling out his hair. His medical records refer to his bald patches as "active post-traumatic alopecia," focusing on the result of the behaviour — *alopecia* means baldness — rather than the cause. But, combine his hair loss with his unusually stubborn behaviour, and it seems likely that Bill was suffering psychological distress — perhaps from an anxiety disorder. If so, it passed under the radar of the medical staff. That was no surprise. The institution was chronically short of staff with medical or psychological training, and staff turnover was high. During Bill's childhood years, no doctor stayed for longer than eighteen months, and more than two dozen psychologists came and went in the psychology department between 1950 and 1965.[6] The handwriting in Bill's medical chart changed with just about every entry, which shows there was little or no continuity of care. On the wards, Bill was just another small body to be fed, clothed, bathed now and then, and taught to take care of his physical needs. His hair pulling was dismissed as merely a quirk.

One person at the institution, however, took note of his psychological distress. She was the author of an unusually detailed occupational therapy report in 1974 that shows Bill's teenage years were troubling.

The writer's five-page report drew on Bill's ward school records from 1968 to 1973, which are otherwise missing from his file, and other documents to which she had access. From 1968 to 1970, she wrote, Bill's school records show he made substantial progress in learning how to speak, dress, and take care of himself. He was mischievous—"can obey simple commands but often chooses not to"; "co-operative except for opening [water] taps at all times"; "runs away for 'fun,' likes being chased"—and insisted on certain routines. However, he made strides in picking up new words: candy, cookie, toast, jam, bread, fork, spoon, cup, milk, gum, and, very proudly, "appy-buhday *too* you." His attention span improved. He learned how to cut his own food, tie his shoes, and button his shirt. He overcame his fear of walking in the snow or on a grassy slope. He took care of a smaller boy in his group spontaneously, showing empathy and concern for others. He understood the concept of taking turns and could follow the right sequence in a group as large as six. Several times, the report's author wrote, he noticed when the date on the calendar needed changing. He enjoyed art class and worked creatively with blocks. He dressed himself proudly in the clothes Mom bought for him, learning how to "mix and match" and keeping his clothes tidy. A note from 1970 said, "great enjoyment displayed in play and work."

In the spring of 1971, Bill moved to a new ward. It was an unhappy move. Mom rarely complained about Bill's care, but this time she

Ontario Hospital School at _____ SMITHS FALLS

PHOTOGRAPHIC RECORD

Case Book No. _____ 2690

Name ____ McKERCHER: William Andrew _____   Admitted ____ February 18 1959

Photograph taken ____ May ____ 19*60*   Photograph taken ____ *1971* ____ 19 ___

Photograph taken ____ *Dec* 19 *76*   Photograph taken ____ *February* ____ 19 ___

1M-69-2847

Bill began pulling out his hair when he was nine or ten, starting with his eyelashes and eyebrows. As these institutional photos show, by the time he was twenty the extent of his hair loss was startling.

apparently did. The institution moved him to a different ward in fairly quick order. In a family survey Mom filled out later that year, she wrote, "I was pleased on my last visit to see our son Bill in East 4C where the whole atmosphere was a vast improvement on his previous ward, W5D. His improved behaviour and interest reflected the change." This was her way of thanking the institution for responding to her complaints about the ward, and reminding them that she found the atmosphere on W5D toxic.

The occupational therapy report skips from 1971 to the spring of 1973. There's no explanation for the gap, but it's clear that Bill did not do well in those years. Instead of adding words to his vocabulary, he lost them. By 1973, he had "practically no spontaneous speech." Instead of proudly wearing his own clothes, he was wearing "institutional clothes" pulled from a bin in the ward with little thought or care. Bill had always been a tease, but now his mischievous nature had taken a mean turn: "very clever at getting other children into trouble and then enjoys the ruckus from a distance." It appears he had also been put to work on the ward: "Mops floors well," the report says.

In March of 1974, he joined the occupational therapy unit known as Granny's House, which promoted free play in a home-like setting and emphasized communication skills. At first, Bill seemed uncomfortable: "Scared to move without permission, does not seem to trust me," the report says. He also displayed some odd mannerisms, including a head shake and a habit of looking around as if seeing things that weren't there. He showed no creativity in playing with the objects in the room. He "seemed very institutionalized, no initiative."

Things improved as the therapist who had written the report worked with him that year. He started to play again and his speech improved. The head shake disappeared. By November, he was wearing his own clothes again and was proud of how he looked. His attention span was longer, and he no longer seemed suspicious or scared. "By now his trust in me is restored," the report concluded. "He is full of enthusiasm arriving at the sessions, he works well." However, "the intense joy in work and play he showed four years ago seems absent."

What happened to Bill between 1970 and 1973 that made him regress so much? Was he abused, neglected, bullied, or mistreated? Was he sexually assaulted? Was he depressed? Did he simply get lost in the crowd? I wish I had an answer, but I don't. His personal file for those years reveals nothing. Nor do the institutional records I examined at the Archives of Ontario. His medical records show he was on antibiotics several times in 1970, once for a cough, three times for an unspecified wound that needed to be dressed—whether an injury or another of his frequent staph infections, it is impossible to say. He had a serious unspecified illness in August of 1972, and a playground injury, again unspecified, put him in the infirmary for two weeks in September of the same year. He had several episodes of vomiting and diarrhea. None of this, however, explains why he sank so low. I have no idea whether he was miserable because he was ill so often, or ill because he was so miserable. I don't know whether the injury that put him in the infirmary was a cause of his unhappiness or a way of escaping the misery of his ward. Again, there's nothing in the record to suggest anyone cared to figure out why.

It was a relief to see that he eventually regained his enthusiasm for life. But how heartbreaking to read that the "intense joy" for learning he felt at one point in his life had been dampened, apparently permanently. He would never get it back, never make the strides in language or creativity he made when he was twelve, thirteen, or fourteen. Succumbing to dullness was the price he paid for institutional life, or at least part of the price. The balance came due when he was thirty-eight.

Chapter 7

"A CENTURY OF **FAILURE** AND **INHUMANITY**"

During the years Bill was shut away inside the hospital school in Smiths Falls, attitudes on the outside toward people like him were changing. This reflected, in part, an expanded and more egalitarian view of citizenship, one that was beginning to recognize the legitimate aspirations and rights of previously marginalized groups. The notion that having a disabled child was a mark of shame for a family—a sign of tainted blood or a punishment from God—was finally fading. So was the idea that children with disabilities should be sent to institutions like hospital schools as a matter of course. Many parents felt integration into community schools would be a better choice for their children. Despite these advances, though, the network of institutions for people with intellectual disabilities continued to grow.

The fledgling parents groups that began popping up after the Second World War coalesced, in the 1950s and 1960s, into increasingly active provincial, national, and international associations, united around the idea of promoting community-based care. The US National Association of Parents and Friends of Mentally Retarded Children, created in 1950, had 119 local chapters in 1952; by 1958 there were 550.[1] In Canada, a number of fast-growing provincial associations came together in 1958 to form the Canadian Association for Retarded Children.[2] These groups began to demand services from government, not as charity but as a right.

The Ontario Association for Retarded Children,[3] founded in 1953 as a lobbying and advocacy group, saw education for children with intellectual disabilities as, in essence, a civil rights issue. Because all taxpayers contribute to the public school system, it argued, all children should have the right to go to school. Ontario's Education Act prohibited public school boards from accepting children whose IQs were less than 50, or one-half the average IQ of 100.[4] The provincial hospital school was the only place where such a child could get an education. An early activist summed up the contradiction in this policy in 1949: "If these children can be taught something at Orillia why cannot a day school be put at their disposal?"[5]

Parents who didn't want to send their children away organized classes on their own. The first one in Ontario opened in 1947 in Kirkland Lake. The province had allowed auxiliary classes for students with lower IQs since the early years of the twentieth century, but teacher Don Frisby believed it was unfair to bar children with IQs below the cutoff of 50 from going to school. He rallied local civic and service club leaders and wrote to Premier George Drew asking for financial support. The department of education came up with a small grant—$2,500 a year for three years—to help support the new class. The Kirkland Lake experiment, which operated out of rented space in a church basement, attracted a lot of positive reaction, both locally and nationally. Classes in other communities followed, funded by donations, staffed by auxiliary teachers, and run in places other than schools.[6] Betty Anglin, a long-time activist and co-author of a 1978 history of the Ontario Association for the Mentally Retarded, described the spirit that inspired those early classes: "Professional educators, social workers and neighbours encouraged parents to find answers to the questions they were now brave enough to ask, e.g. 'why can't my child go to school?' 'why must my child leave home for training?' 'why should I feel excluded from society because my child has a handicap?'"[7]

Under pressure from these parent associations, the province agreed in 1953 to contribute a modest per-student stipend for community schools. The money came with strings, however. The parents groups had to run the classes, no one under eighteen could be charged a fee to attend, and the length of classes had to be between two and three hours a day, no longer or shorter.[8] The length of the school day was increased later on in the 1950s, but younger children—those under twelve—still couldn't go to full-day school. Under those rules, Bill would have had to wait until 1968 to start going to school full-time.

The parent-run classes proved popular and spread quickly. By 1960, the year after Bill moved to Smiths Falls, 1,950 Ontario children with intellectual disabilities were enrolled in sixty-six schools across the province.[9] However, the burden of organizing and staffing the schools still fell on the parent groups. Over the next few years, the province created special education authorities that took over that work, and the amount of funding increased. Finally, at the end of the 1960s, local public school boards took over these programs. This shift raised some new issues: whether to integrate these children into regular classes or create special public school classes, and how many and what kind of aides they needed. But, sending a child with a significant developmental disability to the same public school as everyone else in the neighbourhood went from being a radical—even illegal—act ten years before my brother was born to being business as usual ten years after he was born.

The developments in Canada paralleled—or, more typically, followed—what was going on in the United States. Within months of his election as president, John F. Kennedy appointed a panel of professionals to make recommendations on all aspects of what was then called mental retardation policy. The panel reported back in late 1962 with more than one hundred recommendations. On February 5, 1963, Kennedy announced what he called "a bold new approach" toward helping those with intellectual disabilities and their families, including new programs for maternity and prenatal care, plans to move away from custodial institutions to community-centred agencies, proposals for new research, better special education and training programs, and improved rehabilitation. Kennedy's successor, Lyndon Johnson, created a presidential committee on intellectual impairments that continues to work today.[10]

The year after Kennedy's announcement, the Canadian national health minister, Judy LaMarsh, called a federal-provincial conference on the same issue. Speaker after speaker emphasized the need for and benefits of community care for children with intellectual disabilities and support for their families. Dr. R.O. Jones of Dalhousie University summed up some of the key ideas: "Home and community care is desirable; removal to a foster home or institution should only be carried out for specific purposes and for a limited time."[11] Health care policy is a provincial matter in Canada, so the kind of national initiative promoted by President Kennedy was less evident in the patchwork of Canadian jurisdictions. Nonetheless, it was clear that the tide was turning.

Two key words would occupy the imagination of advocates for children with disabilities over the next few decades: *normalization* and *deinstitutionalization*. Normalization, coined by the head of Sweden's association for children with disabilities in 1959, refers to "letting the mentally retarded obtain an existence as close to normal as possible."[12] In practice, the push for normalization often meant altering the design and operation of residential institutions to make them look and feel less like dormitories or prison ranges, and more like family homes. But normalization quickly gained additional meaning among advocates, especially on this side of the Atlantic. In the institutional setting, they argued, normalization would never be more than window dressing: genuine normalization required getting people out of the institutions and back into the community.

Picking up on this trend, Ontario passed legislation in the 1960s to promote the development of privately owned, government-funded residences that were supposed to look and feel more like homes than hospital schools. The Homes for Retarded Persons program, aimed specifically at people like Bill, was slow to get off the ground, however. Just eight homes were in operation by 1970, and four of those were sponsored by local associations for the mentally retarded.[13] A second type of residence, known as Homes for Special Care, became widespread much more quickly. This program initially targeted psychiatric patients who were not likely to benefit from further treatment, but it soon expanded to include people released from the hospital schools. Meanwhile, sheltered workshops — segregated workplaces run by local associations for the mentally retarded as a way of giving people a chance to do meaningful work — had begun appearing in the late 1950s. By 1970, more than eighty of these workshops were in operation, providing jobs — if not labour rights — to twenty-two hundred people.[14]

But none of this addressed the intractable problem of life in the institutions: How could *anyone* have a "normal" life when they were shut away in a hospital school, isolated from their families, forced to share living spaces with strangers, prevented from casual contact and friendships with the other sex, isolated from the daily routines of either urban or rural life, and treated as though their intellectual condition was some sort of disease?

The solution was to get rid of the institutions.

A spate of critical media reports fed into — and fed on — increasingly critical views of the institutions. One of the earliest exposés, published in the late 1940s, showed photographs of residents at Letchworth Village in Rockland County, NY. Founded in 1911 as a model community, supported by rich donors, and built to look like Thomas Jefferson's Monticello, Letchworth Village presented itself to the world as the best public facility of its kind, a "village of the simple" in the finest sense of the word. It looked great from the outside. The inside, as photographer Irving Haberman revealed, was a different story. His photos of naked, unkempt, and filthy Letchworth Village residents, huddled in sterile day rooms, shocked readers of New York's *PM* newspaper when they appeared in 1946. Two years later, Albert Deutsch reproduced them in a book, *The Shame of the States*, and charged that Letchworth residents were undergoing "euthanasia through neglect."[15]

In the 1960s, reporters from various media outlets turned their attention to Willowbrook on New York City's Staten Island. With six thousand residents, Willowbrook was the largest public institution for people with intellectual disabilities in the United States. When Senator Robert Kennedy made an unannounced visit to Willowbrook in 1965, he found residents "living in filth and dirt, their clothing in rags, in rooms less comfortable and cheerful than the cages in which we put animals in a zoo."[16] A number of journalists filed reports about the problems at the institution, the most famous of them a 1972 exposé by Geraldo Rivera for WABC-TV in New York. The images he filmed — naked residents rolling or lying on the floor, staff stuffing gruel into residents' mouths so quickly the residents choked, filth everywhere — were shocking and disturbing.[17]

A January 6, 1960, column by the *Toronto Star*'s Pierre Berton about conditions at the Ontario Hospital School at Orillia sent shockwaves through the province.[18] "On the last afternoon of 1959," he wrote, "I drove to Orillia with a friend of mine and his 12-year-old son." They were taking the boy back to the hospital school after the Christmas holidays. Berton was shocked by what he saw there: "There are 2,807 others like him, jammed together in facilities which would be heavily taxed if 1,000 patients were removed. More than 900 of them are hived in 70-year-old buildings. There is nowhere else for them to go."

The buildings had peeling paint, leaky roofs, gaping holes in the plaster walls, and pitted floors repaired with plywood and stinking of urine. In the older buildings, the stairwells were fireproofed but the living spaces were not, leading those residents who were the most disabled to be housed in the newer, better fireproofed cottages. The higher-functioning residents lived in the main building, apparently because they'd be better able, theoretically, to escape a fire.

But what really bothered Berton was the overcrowding: "The beds are crammed together, head to head, sometimes less than a foot apart. I counted 90 in a room designed for 70. There are beds on the veranda. There are beds in classrooms. There are beds in the occupational therapy rooms and in the playrooms that can no longer be used for play. On some floors the patients have nowhere to go except out into the corridors."

The bathroom facilities were primitive: "On one floor there is one wash basin to serve 64 persons. On another floor, where the patients sometimes must be bathed twice or three times a day, there is one bathtub for 144 persons—together with three shower outlets and eight toilets." He added, with a tone of disgust, "Prisoners in reformatories have better facilities."

Berton reported that the hospital school was intended for children aged six or older, but that many of its residents were under that age. The waiting list had four thousand names, fifteen hundred of them added in the last year, and Orillia had admitted 196 new patients in 1949 and 310 in 1959. "At the present time they are coming in at the rate of three a day," he wrote. "The hospital loses, by death or discharge, less than half the number it admits annually. And so the terrifying problem builds up year by year."

He concluded that the problem was a lack of attention; governments would rather spend money on eye-catching public projects, and the public preferred to turn a blind eye to the lives of these people. "Remember this," he wrote. "After Hitler fell, and the horrors of the slave camps were exposed, many Germans excused themselves because they said they did not know what went on behind those walls; no one had told them. Well, you have been told about Orillia."

Berton's article caused a sensation. It was so effective, according to his biographer, that the leader of one of the opposition political parties toured the facility the very next day, and declared the conditions "intolerable." In the next Throne Speech, the government promised funds for more facilities.[19]

Other reporters took up the issue. A 1965 *Globe and Mail* article, for example, confronted the twin problems of overcrowding and under-staffing at the Smiths Falls hospital school. "Each day education in this government institution becomes less of a reality and the name 'school' more of a misnomer," reporter Marvin Schiff wrote. The institution had less than half the trained staff it needed, and seven hundred more residents than the two thousand it was built to accommodate. "In such a setting, custody consumes most of the time of the harried staff and any opportunity for treatment or education is a luxury. Staff morale, already at a low ebb, degenerates steadily, but the real victims are the patients—most of them children or adolescents." Wards designed for thirty-six residents had eighty or more, with beds crowding out areas to play. In such confined spaces, bruises, bumps, and scratches were common. And, in one recent case, Schiff reported, an injury had turned deadly when a young boy developed blood poisoning and died. A coroner's jury blamed overcrowding. Schiff quoted Dr. Harold Frank, the superintendent, as saying Smiths Falls had no speech therapists and physiotherapists on staff at the time. Doctors and psychologists came and went, staying only for a few months or a year before moving on. The place had two psychiatrists, two psychologists, and three general practitioners, about half the number needed. It had fifty nurses; it could have used one hundred. Frank sounded frustrated with the situation. He told the reporter Ontario should start a crash program of finding homes in the community for some people with mild impairments, and building group homes for others. He also suggested the province should establish smaller institutions—with up to three hundred residents—in sparsely populated regions. More critically, Frank recommended that the department of education should run those smaller institutions, not the department of health. Ironically, and without using the exact words, he was calling for a variation on the nineteenth-century "boarding school for idiots" model, rather than the custodial institutional model that replaced it.[20]

In October of 1966, the *Globe and Mail* reported that the parents of a boy who had nearly died at Smiths Falls were launching a campaign for a public investigation into the way the hospital schools were run. Their ten-year-old son suffered a ruptured spleen when another boy hit him, and the injury went unnoticed for three days. The parents wanted to know the results of a closed-door inquiry into the incident. According to the newspaper, "They say the hospital schools are so badly understaffed that they cannot provide adequate custodial care, let alone treatment for patients."[21] A few months later, the *Globe and Mail* reported on an accusation from a member of the provincial legislature that "severe and serious overcrowding" was responsible for the "bewildering regularity" of deaths at the Smiths Falls hospital school. New Democrat MPP Stephen Lewis said seven residents, most of them children, had died in accidents at Smiths Falls over the previous four years, including four who drowned. The facility was severely overcrowded, he said, and the professional staff was less than 50 per cent of the required number.[22] In April of 1969, the newspaper reported that thirteen teenagers ran away from the hospital school one Sunday and tried to walk to Ottawa. Four of them wandered back around dinnertime; a police dog found the others huddled in the woods at five a.m. on Monday morning, "frightened, cold and hungry but otherwise unhurt." They were six miles from the institution. The report also noted that a twenty-two-year-old who ran away from Smiths Falls in July of 1966 had drowned, and a sixteen-year-old who had done the same the previous February had died of exposure.[23]

Articles like these dealt with specific incidents, but taken together they pointed to a larger narrative. If the hospital schools couldn't attract and keep enough staff, if they couldn't give residents the health care or education they needed, if the government was failing to provide enough funding to do anything more than keep children in custody, if some of those children were injured or dying, then the time had come to think about why the province persisted in operating these institutions. There had to be a better way.

But it took a tragedy — or, more accurately, two tragedies — to bring about real change.

—

In March 1971, Frederick Elijah Sanderson, a Smiths Falls hospital school resident who had been sent out to do farm work for a local farmer, was found hanging by his neck in a hayloft on his employer's farm. Sanderson was weeks away from his nineteenth birthday. At the time of his death, another former resident who had been sent out to do farm work, Jean Marie Martel, was recuperating in hospital from severe frostbite injuries received while running away from the farm where he had been assigned.[24]

Sanderson's story was tragic on just about every level. After losing both parents, he went into foster care at the age of four and lived in thirteen different foster homes. When he failed grade one for the third time, his local children's aid society sent him to Smiths Falls. He arrived a few years after my brother, in 1962. The institution's experts diagnosed him as having a "low moron level" of intelligence—between a mild and moderate disability. In 1969, after several years at Smiths Falls, the hospital school sent him to live with his brother in Kapuskasing, in northern Ontario. When that didn't work out, his brother sent him back to Smiths Falls. The hospital school then sent him to work for a local farmer. Sanderson would get room and board, $20 a month, and $5 a week in spending money.

Though a social worker from the institution took him to the farm and visited regularly, no one inspected the room he was given in the damp and filthy basement of the farmhouse. Less than a month after moving in, Sanderson said he was unhappy and wanted to return to the institution. He was homesick, the social worker said, and didn't like farm work. Sanderson went back to Smiths Falls several times for visits or medical appointments, but the institution kept returning him to the farm. He refused to go back at least twice in 1970, but each time the institution sent him back anyway, after a few days or weeks. The last time anyone from the institution saw him was just before Christmas in 1970. A few days before what should have been the next visit by a social worker, in March of 1971, the farmer's son found Sanderson hanging from the rafters. The son went to get his father, who then called the police. The police arrived an hour later. The farmer showed them to the hayloft, where Sanderson was still hanging. Neither father nor son had thought of cutting him down.

The coroner's jury ruled the death a suicide. It also issued a statement deploring "the lack of professional supervision afforded the deceased in this case from the time of his first placement until the time of his death," and recommending both tighter screening of potential placements for former residents and better monitoring of how a placement was working out.

Days later, news broke in the Ottawa newspapers about another former hospital school resident, twenty-four-year-old Jean Marie Martel. Martel had been found walking along a country road on a bitterly cold February day, two weeks before Sanderson's death, with his nose, ears, and fingers frostbitten. He was taken to a hospital and diagnosed with gangrene on all the fingertips of his right hand, and three of the fingers on his left hand.

Martel's story was similar in some ways to Sanderson's. He had no father, and was raised by his grandparents until their deaths sometime in 1961, when he was about fourteen. Martel then moved in with his mother, but landed within a year at Smiths Falls, where his intelligence level was assessed as "high imbecile," or moderately impaired. Over the next six years he received no schooling, but did learn how to speak English reasonably well. (His first language was French.) In 1967, when Martel was twenty, the institution sent him out to work on a farm in nearby Richmond, Ontario. The family running the farm agreed to give him room and board, and $40 a month in pay. The rehabilitation officer who dropped him off left Martel with two phone numbers, his mother's and the institution's, and told him he could leave or stay. The numbers were of little use to Martel, who did not know how to dial a telephone.

Things went well for the first few months, and the institution formally discharged Martel from care in April 1968, when he was twenty-one. But relations between Martel and the family soured. Martel ran away and refused to return to the farm. His mother didn't want him to move back in with her, and since he had been officially discharged from the hospital school, the rehabilitation officer didn't want to take him back to Smiths Falls. Instead, he moved Martel to a different farm.

Again, the first few months went well. But, in the winter of 1969, Martel got frostbite on his fingers. He became morose, grumbled about the work, and began to wander away from the farm. The farmer complained that Martel ate too much and worked too little, and locked Martel out of the house now and then to stop him from raiding the fridge. One day, Martel exposed himself to a couple of young girls. The farmer, furious, attacked him. He said later, "I kicked him in the arse—what would you do?" Martel stayed on at the farm, but the farmer had no more time for him.

In the summer of 1970, Martel hurt his hand in a truck door, losing the tip of a finger. He also began soiling his pants. The farmer's wife wouldn't let him into the house until he cleaned himself up, which he did in an unheated garage next to the house. That was acceptable in the summer, but cold work in the winter. On February 4, 1971, he wandered away from the farm. It was a bitterly cold day, and he had no gloves. The farmer found him in Richmond and took him back to the farm. Martel wandered away again on the eleventh and the eighteenth, the final time after being locked out of the house. This time another farmer found him, but Martel refused point blank to go back to the farm. He was taken to hospital that night, where the doctors discovered gangrene, a potentially life-threatening condition. Because he had nowhere else to go, he stayed at the hospital for four weeks. Eventually, his mother came and got him.

No charges were laid. But with two sensational incidents of apparent abuse, one of them leading to suicide, and amid a growing chorus of people calling for change in how Ontario took care of people like Martel and Sanderson, Ontario's new health minister, Albert (Bert) Lawrence, realized he had to do something. Lawrence appointed a well-known Toronto lawyer, Walter Williston, to investigate these incidents and the institutional context in which they occurred, and to recommend how the province could do a better job.

The result, delivered in August of 1971, was a comprehensive, critical assessment not just of the Sanderson and Martel cases, but of the entire system the province had built for taking care of people with intellectual disabilities.

Williston began his report by setting out a "statement of principles and objectives."[25] Every individual, regardless of ability, has a basic human right to "such assistance, protection, opportunity and shelter as will enable him to take his place as a contributing member of the community and to ensure him a decent standard of living so that he can walk through life with dignity," he wrote. As much as possible, this help should take place in the family and the community. The goal should be to give each individual the "maximum degree of normalcy," to foster their healthy and happy development as a total person. According to the report, the best ways to achieve these objectives were to put one government department in charge of planning, coordinating, programming, budgeting, and financing the services people needed and, at the same time, to promote regional self-sufficiency in delivering those services.

All too often, Williston observed, admission to an institution was seen as an end solution for children with intellectual disabilities, their parents, and society. By continuing to rely on large institutions, where the emphasis was on custody rather than rehabilitation, Ontario had failed to meet its obligations. "I suggest that a century of failure and inhumanity in the large multi-purpose residential hospitals for the retarded should, in itself, be enough to warn of the inherent weakness in the system and inspire us to look for some better solution," he wrote.[26] The province should phase out the big institutions as quickly as possible, he urged, and build a new system emphasizing community care in their place.

The report contained a detailed examination of who was being housed in the provincial system. Williston wrote that 11,300 Ontario residents with intellectual disabilities were living in a range of provincially funded institutions in 1971.[27] More than half of them — sixty-five hundred individuals — were in facilities owned and operated by the health department's mental retardation branch, which included the three large Ontario hospital schools and eight smaller or more specialized centres. Another thirteen hundred had moved, over the previous three years, into so-called Homes for Special Care that were designed for people with intellectual or psychiatric disabilities who would not benefit from treatment. The rest of the residents were divided among a range of provincially funded facilities, some of them operated by local associations, which included special wards in psychiatric hospitals, community residences, children's boarding residences, and sanatoriums.

Using minimum standards for ward staff set by the American Association for Mental Deficiency, Williston found that the three biggest provincial institutions were understaffed by between 24 per cent and 29 per cent. In raw numbers, Smiths Falls had 2,070 residents and 782 ward staff, but needed at least 1,055 staff members to meet minimum staffing levels. The Cedar Springs institution, at Blenheim in what's now the Municipality of Chatham-Kent, had 937 residents and 354 ward staff, and needed at least 469 more staff members. Orillia had 1,857 residents in its main facility and another 358 in its Muskoka unit in Gravenhurst, which had opened in the mid-1960s to ease congestion at the institution. The main facility had 653 staff members, 257 below the minimum standard. The Muskoka unit, with 138 staff, was 58 members below the minimum standard.[28]

While staffing levels were better in the smaller facilities, wrote Williston, many of these facilities had other problems. The Midwestern Regional Children's Centre in rural Palmerston, between Toronto and Lake Huron, was just six years old but its residents included thirty adults who had been admitted as children, and now had nowhere else to go. "There are essentially no programs for these adults," Williston wrote.[29] The Adult Occupational Centre at Edgar, a residential centre that prepared young adults and older adolescents to return to the community, was "a fine concept" but had a "major defect": Edgar had been built on the site of a former military radar station near Lake Simcoe, miles away from the nearest town, so the people living there had no actual experience of living in a community.[30] At the men's institution in Aurora, near Toronto, which had opened in the early 1950s to ease overcrowding at Orillia, residents lived in what the administrators called "cottage units." These units were, in fact, the upper floors of a converted boys' school, and residents slept "virtually elbow to elbow." Despite attempts to modify and redecorate the building, Williston declared that "the facility is obsolete."[31] The facility at Cobourg, on Lake Ontario east of Toronto, was meant to provide training and rehabilitation programs for women with mild to moderate impairments so they could move back into the community. Several of its residents, however, were elderly and unable to move about, and between sixty and seventy of them had psychiatric illnesses, which disrupted the training and rehabilitation programs.[32]

Williston's critique of the institutions that existed in Ontario echoed and reinforced all the complaints parents, teachers, medical staff, experts on institutions, advocates for deinstitutionalization, and support groups had been voicing for years. These included the fact that, instead of helping individuals reach their full potential, life in these institutions forced residents to function far below their development capacity. Williston cited overcrowded wards; "dull, monotonous and impersonal" living conditions; limits on private possessions; little or no personal privacy, including in the bathrooms; almost complete segregation of the sexes; unnecessarily locked wards; weakened contacts between residents and their families; isolation; a continuation of the traditional emphasis on custody, rather than training or rehabilitation; and a chronic shortage of the kind of experts the institutions needed. "There is always an insufficient number of physicians; psychiatrists; dentists; psychologists; occupational, physical and speech therapists; nurses; social workers and other skilled professionals," he wrote. Remote locations isolated residents from researchers and universities, but geographic isolation was only part of the problem: "The difficulty of interesting trained personnel in working with the retarded in isolated institutions is compounded by the comparatively low salaries and other restrictions professional persons feel are imposed by governmental personnel practices."[33]

Former residents found it difficult to navigate life on the outside. The longer someone lives in the institution, Williston wrote, the harder it is to function in the broader world. People who left the institution were stigmatized as former residents, while institutional life inhibited the kinds of social contacts a resident needed to adjust to life into the community. "In other words, to rehabilitate the retarded person who has lived the better part of his life in an institution is almost impossible."[34]

Williston believed there was a role for institutions, but that it should be limited to providing nursing or medical care, behaviour modification, crisis intervention, training for parents, and medical research. He speculated that reorienting the institutions towards this kind of work could cut their populations by 60 per cent.[35] At the same time, he indicated that families should get the financial, social, educational, and personal support they needed to keep their children with intellectual disabilities at home.

This should not, he stressed, mean keeping them at home forever. As children became adults, he thought they should have the chance to move into a community residence near home and a sheltered workshop. Williston envisioned "a large number of small facilities" spread across the province, integrated with the educational, recreational, and commercial parts of the community. These residences would look and feel like private houses or apartments, not institutions, and they would take a number of forms — specialized long-term residential houses, apartments and cooperatives, halfway houses to prepare people for independent living, and specialized nursing homes for those who need chronic care. He proposed a variety of facilities for children whose families were unable to care for them fully, such as foster homes, residences for those who couldn't be placed in foster homes, temporary boarding houses, or short-term residential treatment centres. These facilities would be part of what he called "social care," where communities would have the responsibility to provide families and individuals with all the educational, recreational, employment, medical, dental, psychological, and social services they needed.[36]

As the tragic cases of Sanderson and Martel had shown, the existing system was broken. But, in a tightly written 113 pages, Williston offered a way to rebuild it.

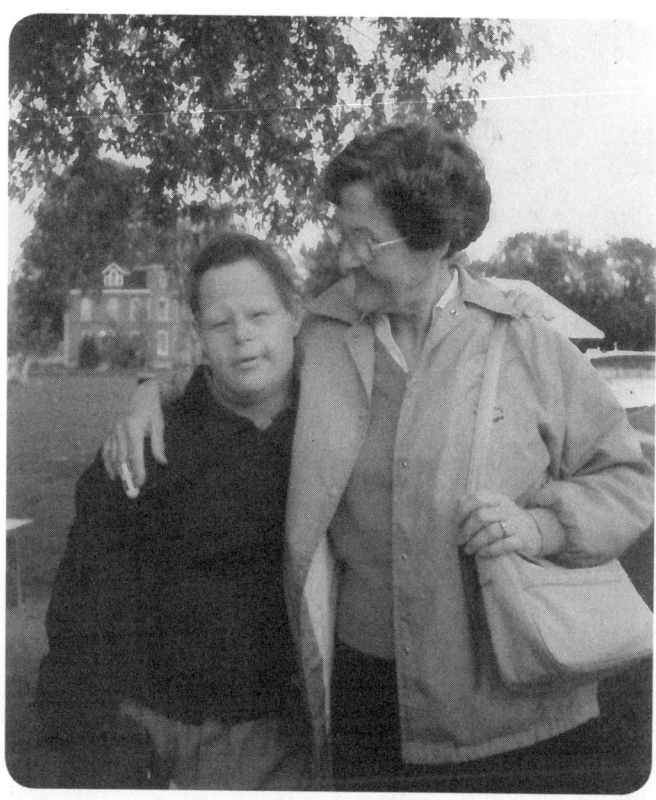

By the time Dad took this photo of Mom and Bill in the early
1980s, the government was talking about shutting down
the institutions. My parents opposed the idea.

—

Perhaps it was the timing, coinciding with the growing movement to
normalize and deinstitutionalize people like my brother Bill. Perhaps
it was the care with which Williston, a respected outsider who had no
personal stake in the issue, went about his work. Or perhaps it was a
magical combination of common sense and an appeal to our better selves.
In any case, the Williston report received an enthusiastic reception.

Almost immediately, Health Minister Lawrence announced that the
population of the three big Ontario institutions would be cut by 60 per
cent over the next five years. The minister also promised to redirect

funds from the institutions to residences and services in the community. "I can't see any recommendation I would quarrel with," he told a press conference.[37] The leaders of the Liberal and New Democratic parties both announced that they agreed with the report's recommendations. Wolf Wolfensberger, a leading figure in the move toward deinstitutionalization who was working in Toronto at the National Institute on Mental Retardation at the time, offered his fulsome support. "In the Williston report I found most of the progressive thought on this topic that is available from across the world," he wrote to the *Globe and Mail*. "If Ontario rises even partly to the challenge of the Williston report, it will become a leader of enlightenment in human services in North America."[38]

In 1972, Bill Davis, the premier of Ontario, reorganized his cabinet and put Robert Welch in charge of social development policy. Instead of supervising one ministry, Welch's job as provincial secretary for social development was to work with a half-dozen ministries that all had something to do with social services, including those for people with intellectual impairments. Welch produced a green paper the next year that set out an "explicit, detailed commitment to a reorientation of policy toward community care."[39] The report's introduction started with a quote from Williston: "If a mentally retarded child is to be provided with the assistance he needs to face the problems of adult life and is given the opportunity to develop to his ultimate potential, he must at all times be given the greatest possible degree of participation in life." Welch picked up the theme, writing, "It follows that, wherever feasible, services should be provided in a community setting as an alternative to institutionalization."[40] He acknowledged that moving people from institution to community would be neither cheap nor easy, but stressed that these difficulties could and should be overcome.

Over the next few years, the province took up the challenge of rebuilding the hospital school system. The most significant decision made was to transfer responsibility for the institutions from the ministry in charge of health to the Ministry of Community and Social Services. This was not simply a bureaucratic shuffle. Repudiating the long-standing medical model of institutional care, Welch believed a government department tailored to providing social welfare and a broad range of community services was a better choice to take care of the needs of people with intellectual disabilities.

The names of the institutions were changed: the one at Smiths Falls became the Rideau Regional Centre, the one at Orillia was renamed the Huronia Regional Centre, and the one at Cedar Springs became the Southwestern Regional Centre. Again, these changes were not merely symbolic. They reflected, at least on an aspirational level, a fundamental change in the province's approach to care.

Part of the incentive behind the movement to community and social services was financial. Williston had not done an analysis of what community care would cost or save the province in his report, but he provided some data showing that hospital school care was much more expensive than other forms of care. More crucially, the province was eager to take advantage of a fairly new federal program, the Canada Assistance Plan, which reimbursed 50 per cent of provincial spending on social assistance. When institutional residents were transferred to the community and social services ministry, they became eligible for this money; if they stayed as patients of facilities run by the Ontario health ministry, they did not qualify. In his history of institutional care in Ontario, Harvey Simmons writes that it was hard to know whether the desire to get access to the federal money prompted the transfer of patients, or whether the move would have happened anyway. He speculates it was the latter: "The fact remains that in Canada, the US and in Great Britain, there was a shared feeling among those interested in and responsible for mental retardation policy that the time had come to reduce the size of large institutions, and to establish some kind of community service program for mentally retarded people."[41]

The rhetoric of deinstitutionalization outpaced the reality of its implementation, however, and the system proved resistant to change. The big institutions did not shrink by 60 per cent within five years, as the health minister promised, but declined far more slowly — by about

30 per cent between 1971 and 1977. At Huronia, the number of residents dropped from 1,857 to 1,254, while the population at Smiths Falls fell from 2,070 to 1,334, and the Cedar Springs population went from 937 to 805. At the same time, the government also opened a handful of additional, smaller institutions in the first half of the 1970s, around the same time as the big institutions were starting to shrink. When you add in the populations of those new facilities, the decline in the number of people living in institutions is less sharp: about 9 per cent. It seems that part of the promised reduction in the sizes of the big institutions was achieved by moving people to the smaller ones.[42]

Nonetheless, by the middle of the 1970s, the tide that swept kids like my brother into the institutions had turned. Over the next decades, the numbers of institutional residents would continue to decline as government and institution officials began to move people, one by one, out of places like Huronia and the Rideau Regional Centre and into group homes, supported-living apartments, nursing homes, or smaller institutions.

One of the people they tried to move was Bill.

Chapter 8

"ONLY WHEN HE BECOMES MORE ADVANCED"

After the Ministry of Community and Social Services took over Ontario's institutions in the early 1970s, the volume of paperwork in Bill's file exploded. More paperwork did not always translate into meaningful information, however. Scores of forms appeared to be filled out largely for the sake of filling out forms. A seemingly endless stream of program reports, for example, set goals like "Bill will maintain independence in tooth-brushing skills" or "in the area of showering." Each form then rated how well he did meeting those goals. Month after month after month, someone ticked boxes or gave Bill scores out of a hundred—or, bizarrely, sometimes out of two hundred—on the simple acts of daily life.

But within the pile of paper is a narrative about the trajectory Bill's life would take as he grew from teenager to adult—specifically, about whether (or when) he would leave the Rideau Regional Centre in Smiths Falls.

In March of 1972, the centre sent Mom and Dad a family survey. It had a dozen questions, most of them about the level and type of contact they wanted with Bill. The completed survey, filled out by Mom, is in Bill's file. She asked for written reports about him four times a year—the other options were once a month, every six months, once a year, or only on request—and said she would visit him once a month except during the winter. She said the family was not interested in having Bill come to Ottawa for home visits. The sixth question asked, "Do you wish to commence discussions with us as to returning your child to suitable accommodation in your community. i.e. community residence, approved boarding home etc.?" Mom could have ticked a box saying she preferred not to discuss it at all, or a box saying she would like to talk about moving Bill back home with the family. Instead, she ticked the box expressing interest in discussing community accommodation but penned a condition in the margin: "only when he becomes more advanced."

That phrase gnaws at me.

Read literally, it suggests my parents believed that Bill *would* become "more advanced"—advanced enough, eventually, to move out of the institution and into a home in their community. But everything they knew about institutional life by that time—from the thoughtful critique laid out in the Williston report to the negative media reports to the evidence before their eyes of their son's constricted life—told them that wasn't likely to happen. By 1972, it was glaringly obvious that the old promise of "progress and happiness" had not been fulfilled, at least not for Bill. At sixteen, he was losing words, not gaining them. He had become suspicious of people he once trusted. He had given up trying to wear his own clothes, and was fading into the woodwork in institutional garb. He was pulling out his hair. He was living in one big, crowded ward after another, wards where a small and chubby teenager—his medical record lists his adult height as either 4'9" or 4'11"—could easily get lost, bullied, or abused without anyone doing anything about it. So, it's hard for me to believe that Mom and Dad were genuinely convinced that Bill would become "more advanced" at Smiths Falls.

I suspect that what they really meant was "only *if* he becomes more advanced." And, because they had no expectations that this could happen, it was a way of saying no to the idea of moving Bill out of the institution without actually saying no. They might have told themselves the condition they set was a way of keeping Bill safe from the threats and dangers of the wider world, but it was also a way of keeping Bill at a distance from their own lives and our life as a family.

Regardless of how my parents felt, part of the institution's mandate by this time was to move residents into other, hopefully better, living situations. Bill's file contains a decade's worth of "review/transfer out" forms starting in 1978, along with other correspondence running into the 1990s, assessing his readiness to leave the institution and where he might go. The "review/transfer out" forms have a slew of numerical rankings on a number of arcane scales, but the critical one is near the bottom, setting a five-year goal for Bill. These documents make for surreal reading.

The official who filled out the 1978 form, written when Bill was twenty-two, struck through the "transfer out" part of the "review/transfer out" heading—a pretty clear signal that the people in charge didn't think he was ready to leave. The five-year goal it set for Bill was living in a "core residence," presumably the Rideau Regional Centre or another institution like it, or a "special support home." There are two versions of the 1979 form, both bearing the same date. One has exactly the same editing of the heading as the 1978 form, and sets exactly the same goal. The other says Bill would be ready to move to more independent living arrangements in four years. The 1980 form says Bill was eligible for transfer "immediately" to a more independent living arrangement in an unspecified core residence, again most probably somewhere like the Rideau Regional Centre. That fall, however, Bill's name appeared on a list of adult residents being considered for transfer to group homes in Brockville, on the St. Lawrence River south of Smiths Falls. This was a mistake. A few weeks later Bill's name came off the list.

In March of 1981, Bill moved to an independent living unit within the Rideau Regional Centre. The "review/transfer out" form for that year says he'd be eligible for a transfer of some unspecified sort within one year. There are two versions of the 1982 form: one says he would be ready for more independent living in two years; the other version is incomplete. There is no 1983 form. By 1984, the time frame for a move was back up to five years, and the recommended type of housing for Bill was a "special support home (for psychosocial problems)." It was a five-year time frame again in 1985, though this time the form recommends a group home. Both the 1986 and 1987 forms set the time frame for a move at two years out, and indicate the preferred form of housing should be a special support home for people with psychosocial problems.

In the spring of 1987, Bill was identified as a potential candidate for placement in a family home in Ottawa through the Ottawa and District Association for the Mentally Retarded. Bill's case manager at Smiths Falls and the coordinator of the Ottawa program met with Bill to talk about the placement. It did not go well. "Mr. McKercher adamantly stated his refusal to leave Rideau Regional Centre and ended the interview by refusing to answer questions," says a memo about the meeting. I burst out laughing when I read that memo. Bill couldn't say much, but he certainly knew how to say "No!", and it sounds like he said it vigorously. "Mr. McKercher's name has been withdrawn from the list of potential candidates for family home placement," the memo adds. In August, the case manager had another talk with Bill about moving. The note on that conversation reads "Billy indicated to me that he did not wish to leave the centre at this time." Again, this made me laugh. Bill probably just roared "No!", folded his arms across his chest, and refused to say anything more.

In 1988, the time frame for Bill's move out of the Smiths Falls facility was down to six months. The records then skip to 1991, when the institution sent a bunch of documents about Bill to the behaviour management program of the Ottawa Children's Aid Society. In August of 1992, the institution sent a note to the government indicating that Bill "is being considered for discharge," and asking for a social insurance certificate. The card was sent to him on September 25, with a request for him to sign it as soon as possible. This was, of course, impossible. Bill did not know how to write.

The forms stop at this point. In the end, none of this amounted to anything.

—

I had no idea Bill was ever considered for a move to a group, family, or special support home in Ottawa until I got his file; nor did my sister and brother. We also have no idea why the move didn't take place. Aside from Bill's negative reaction to the idea, the documents in his file give no conclusive answers. At the risk of reading too deeply between the lines, though, it seems a number of factors kept Bill at Rideau Regional.

For one, there's no escaping the fact that as an adult, Bill's intellectual impairment was severe. He had attended school at the institution for many years, where, in Mom's view, "he progressed as far as he was capable—which wasn't far." The school at Rideau Regional didn't hand out conventional report cards, but completed reports on the skills he had obtained and what he would work on next. Two examples suffice to convey the state of Bill's intellectual development. The 1976 report describes Bill as "a very friendly exuberant boy who enjoys school. He participates in all areas of the school program. He recognizes his name and similarities in numbers, colours, and shapes. He likes to keep busy and his skills in tracing, colouring, pasting, and cutting are improving." Bill was twenty years old when this report was written. The 1979 report says he could match colours and could name blue, red, brown, and yellow "with some help." This comment triggered a memory of Bill when he was still living at home, happily playing with a colouring book and crayons. He used to call blue "boo"—it was his favourite colour, which explains why it was also his nickname—and yellow "lalo," and you couldn't trick him into saying something "lalo" was "boo." But here he was, twenty years after moving into a hospital school, still being taught the names of colours. The report says he could, however, identify and match a square, circle, triangle, and heart. He was "being exposed to number symbols" and to "the concepts" of one to ten. He could recognize his own name. He was aware of the weather. He had a good sense of rhythm and could stop and start at the correct time in rhythm band. That summer, he took part in a six-week vocabulary learning program, during which he learned to "verbally name" two new words and "identify" three more.

I've often wondered just how much of Bill's impairment was due to Down syndrome and how much to decades of institutional life. A 2018 study found that most Americans with Down syndrome could walk by twenty-five months of age, speak reasonably well by the age of twelve, and maintain personal hygiene by the time they are thirteen. By the age of thirty-one, 49 per cent could read reasonably well and 46 per cent could write reasonably well.[1] Bill met the walking and personal hygiene milestones, but not the others. Had he grown up at home with other verbal children, or gone to a regular public school and had the help of an aide, how well would he have learned to speak? He already had some words as a toddler, and he certainly was capable of learning more. At times during his childhood years at Rideau Regional, in fact, he did. Intensive speech therapy from early childhood on probably could have made a huge difference, but Rideau Regional was chronically short of speech therapists and other specialists. His speech training, like every other part of his education, was at best hit and miss, and without reinforcement, his words disappeared. At one point, someone at Rideau Regional taught him a bit of sign language, an inventive approach to helping someone who was basically non-verbal to communicate. His favourite sign was the one for Santa Claus, which looks like someone stroking a beard, and he remembered it forever. Perhaps intensive sign-language training might have expanded his ability to communicate enormously. He never got that training. All I know is that while he understood just about everything people said to him, his adult vocabulary was limited to a few words and short phrases, uttered in a guttural voice. He never learned to write his name. He never learned numbers. He knew that people traded money for things—a lesson that was reinforced when he was caught shoplifting batteries for his Walkman one day—but he had little idea how to use money. He could not dial a telephone or speak to someone at the other end. He could get on and off a bus—in fact, he loved riding on the bus or in a car—but he could not follow a public transit timetable. He was able to get around the institution grounds on his own, but he could not read a street sign. Wherever he lived, he'd need a lot of help.

He also had some medical conditions that needed careful attention.

In May of 1977, a cleaner found him face down on the floor, twitching and unresponsive, apparently in the midst of a seizure. Afterward, Bill complained of a headache, and was sleepy and lethargic. He was diagnosed with epilepsy. This diagnosis was based entirely on the fact that he'd had a probable seizure. His doctors sent him for a brain scan and a spinal tap, but Bill refused to lie still during the procedure despite being heavily sedated. His doctors put him on a daily dose of phenobarbital, which is inexpensive and effective, and it worked insofar as he didn't have another seizure. Phenobarbital is a barbiturate, and its major side effect is to make the person taking it sleepy. In children, it can interfere with learning and cause behaviour problems. Because of side effects like these, doctors usually consider weaning a patient off anticonvulsant drugs if one or two years go by without a seizure. Sometimes that technique doesn't work, but in many other cases, the seizures go into a kind of remission, and the patient no longer needs the drug.

Five years after his seizure, and with no others reported, Bill was still on phenobarbital. Mom sent a note to his doctor asking why. The doctor replied that it was controlling seizures: "Unless this is posing a problem in some other way I would recommend that this be continued indefinitely." Indefinite barbiturate treatment for someone who'd had a single seizure five years ago seemed like using a sledgehammer to swat a fly, but Mom reluctantly accepted the answer.

What she probably didn't know was that prescribing anticonvulsants like phenobarbital was an all-too-common practice at Smiths Falls and other institutions like it in the mid-1970s. More than 40 per cent of residents were taking tranquilizers—some of them two or more different kinds at a time—and almost one-third were taking anticonvulsants, according to a government-commissioned study reported in the *Globe and Mail*. The study's author, Queen's University psychiatrist Dr. Jun-bi Tu, found that many residents of the Ontario institutions were walking around drooling, twitching, restless, dopey, or constipated from over-medication. "I'd estimate no more than 50 per cent of the medication we prescribe is medically necessary," Dr. Tu said. He attributed much of the problem to a shortage of psychiatrists working in the institutions. This meant that general practitioners with little specialized knowledge were dispensing powerful drugs, and perhaps causing permanent damage. The *Globe and Mail* article also quotes Dr. Bruce McCreary, chairman of a six-member committee on drug use inside the institutions, as saying the biggest problem was polypharmacy, or the simultaneous use of multiple drugs to treat one or more problems, which can raise the possibility of harmful drug interactions. He also pointed to a worrisome tendency to keep a resident on a drug much longer than necessary. McCreary didn't want to be overly critical of the doctors working in these institutions, however. "The doctor has to see one hundred to two hundred disturbed patients on an ongoing basis. It's just not possible in an institutional environment to investigate each individual intensively," he said. "The workload is too much, the knowledge is inadequate and the training is inadequate."[2]

Three more years passed, and Bill was still on daily phenobarbital.

Mom went to a "long-term planning" conference for him in February of 1985. She used the occasion to ask about his medication, complaining that she had been unable to learn exactly what he was taking, how much, and why. The institution agreed to send Bill to a neurologist in May for an assessment. He concluded that, because Bill had not had a seizure for close to eight years, he should be weaned off the phenobarbital. The medical staff at Smiths Falls ignored that advice. The neurologist made the same recommendation six months later, in October, when he saw Bill for a follow-up visit. "I had thought that we were going to reduce this by 15 mg every two months until he was off this," he wrote. "I see no reason not to do this and would like to see him again when he is off medication." Again, his advice fell on deaf ears. After seeing Bill a third time, in December, the doctor wrote, somewhat testily, "I do not understand why the medication has not been reduced as I suggested, by 15 mg every two months until he is off."

The process of cutting Bill's dose finally began in 1986 and lasted until November. He was fine — he had no more seizures. But a curious note on one of the blood tests to check his phenobarbital levels in 1981 hinted at another medical issue: "Hep B positive to be written on lab. Sorry." Over the coming years, Bill's hepatitis B status would prove to be a much more serious problem than the casual tone of this note implied.

Bill also had hypothyroidism, or an under-performing thyroid gland, which is a fairly common condition for people with Down syndrome. It can have serious consequences, however, because the hormones released by the thyroid affect just about every other part of the body. The main symptoms of an underactive thyroid are fatigue, weight gain, mood swings, and lethargy. In someone like Bill, who was overweight and slow-moving to begin with and had spent close to nine years taking a daily barbiturate, an underactive thyroid wouldn't be easy to detect without specialized blood tests. I have no idea how long he had the problem before it was diagnosed in 1988. The treatment is simple and effective — a daily pill of synthetic thyroid hormones — but someone would have to supervise his medication to make sure Bill took it.

Finally, Bill had developed some psychological or behavioural problems. He moved in 1981 to a behaviour management section in his ward, although his records do not explain why other than to say he was "disturbed." Behaviour management units had attracted public attention in the mid to late 1970s, following news reports of staff using devices similar to cattle prods on children, including an eleven-year-old girl at the Southwestern Regional Centre (the former Cedar Springs facility).[3] The girl and a dozen others like her injured themselves, and the electrical device was an attempt to stop that behaviour, according to the report. Bill wasn't like that, but he pulled out his own hair, he was stubborn, and he sometimes misbehaved in public. If Bill was having fun, everyone within hearing range knew it — he'd hoot and shout and laugh and whack strangers on the head; he'd burp and laugh at how hilarious burping sounded, then try to burp again. If Bill was unhappy or feeling anxious about a change in his schedule or simply didn't want to do something he was asked to do, he'd roar or whine or moan or act up, and on at least one occasion, on a day away from the institution, he faked a seizure. In addition, he operated on what one counsellor called "Bill time," which had nothing to do with clocks.

A 1982 report summarized his behavioural problems this way: "has a fear of change, i.e. going downtown; Billy is very slow and habitually late or never arrives for programs; lacking in motivation; can be stubborn at times." The institution put him on something called a token economy program, where he earned tokens for behaviour the institution wanted to encourage and lost tokens if he misbehaved. He could exchange the tokens later for something he wanted. An undated memo in the Archives of Ontario setting out guidelines for behaviour management programs included tokens on a list of behaviour "reinforcers" that also included food treats, privileges, social approval, comforts, and special activity. Chillingly, the same memo set out the rules for using "aversive stimuli" like loud noises, drugs, and electric shock, and stipulated that all electrical equipment using line sources of power "had to be hydro inspected."[4]

Over the years, Bill's counsellors worked with him on how to behave in a store or a restaurant or at a hockey game, with mixed results. Sometimes, he could be talked into better behaviour, like the family day at the institution when Mary asked him to be quiet so Mom could listen to the speeches. Bill, who was bored and wanted to leave, considered Mary's request, nodded, and said, "Okay." Sometimes, though, he could not be convinced to behave, like the day he had a full-scale meltdown in a shoe store because Mom wanted to get him new shoes. She left an apologetic note and money for new shoes with the staff at Rideau Regional. After getting stuck in an elevator at the institution for an hour in 1983, Bill resisted going into other elevators and made sure the world knew how strongly he objected to them. He didn't trust escalators either, and he hated going up and down stairs. His periodic clinical assessments for the early 1990s describe his behaviour disorder simply as "disturbed."

His medical records for 1991-93 add a small nuance: "(Disturbed) Unco-operative."

Another portion of his file, however, sheds some light on the nature of his disturbance. Bill and a group of other Rideau Regional residents were part of a study on dementia and adults with Down syndrome. The psychologist conducting the research theorized that symptoms of obsessive-compulsive disorder were a precursor to dementia or Alzheimer's disease in middle-aged people with the genetic condition. A psychometrist took Bill through the psychologist's compulsive behaviour checklist for people with intellectual disabilities in February 1995. The result was shockingly high. The report, signed by the psychometrist and a senior psychologist at Rideau Regional and dated two months later, said Bill exhibited compulsive behaviour in all five categories examined and displayed sixteen of twenty-five possible compulsions. "This is the highest score that has been obtained on this test, so far, in this facility."

Bill insisted, for example, that objects had to be arranged a certain way and in a particular spot. He needed to sit in *this* chair, not *that* chair. He assigned chairs to everyone else in the room and got upset if someone sat at any place other than the assigned seat. His eating habits were rigid: he had to empty every glass and dish even if he wasn't hungry, and lick every piece of cutlery and every plate. It could take him an hour and a half to finish a full-course meal. On the day the psychometrist evaluated him, "it was evident that he was not feeling well yet he forced himself to eat all his meal and would let no one remove it until each dish or glass was empty," the report said. "He had to stuff it all in even though his actions indicated he was full. At one point he stopped to bang his head on the table when he realized he still had one more dish of food to finish eating."

It took him ages, and several stops and starts, to load his dishes in the dishwasher. He tapped walls, floors, and doors on his way to and from work. When it was time for a bath, he got "stuck" undressing, taking off a sock and putting it on again and taking it off and putting it back on until someone prompted him to take the other sock off. "He will also put only one foot in the tub, then take it out, then put it back in until this too can be interrupted by staff," the report said. "He also insists on putting his head under water at least five times before his bath is complete." He scratched his back and buttocks compulsively when he used the urinal, leaving long marks. He stared at himself in the mirror, so much so that the counsellors wouldn't let him have one in his room. According to the report, his counsellors estimated that his compulsive behaviours took up between one and three hours a day: "Not only do they interfere with his normal routine but his social activities and his relationships with others suffered because of his frustrations with himself and others who attempt to intervene." The psychologist wrote that Bill had a long history of this kind of behaviour, and he was not convinced it was linked to the onset of dementia. Instead, he recommended that Bill start taking an antidepressant known to work well for obsessive-compulsive disorder, or OCD.

It's hard to know what to make of this report. OCD is an intractable and deeply frustrating variation of anxiety. People who suffer from it feel unreasonable thoughts and fears, and cope with them through repetitive, compulsive behaviours. "You may try to ignore or stop your obsessions, but that only increases your distress and anxiety," says an overview on the disorder on the Mayo Clinic's website. "Ultimately, you feel driven to perform compulsive acts to try to ease your stress. Despite efforts to ignore or get rid of bothersome thoughts or urges, they keep coming back. This leads to more ritualistic behavior—the vicious cycle of OCD."[5] According to *Psychology Today*, "Often the person carries out the behaviors to get rid of the obsessive thoughts, but this only provides temporary relief. Not performing the obsessive rituals can cause great anxiety."[6]

If Bill was as seriously affected as the psychological report suggested —at the top of the scale for OCD, according to the checklist—he must have been a stew of anxieties and frustrations. His long history of "stubborn" behaviour suddenly makes sense, and so does his hair pulling.

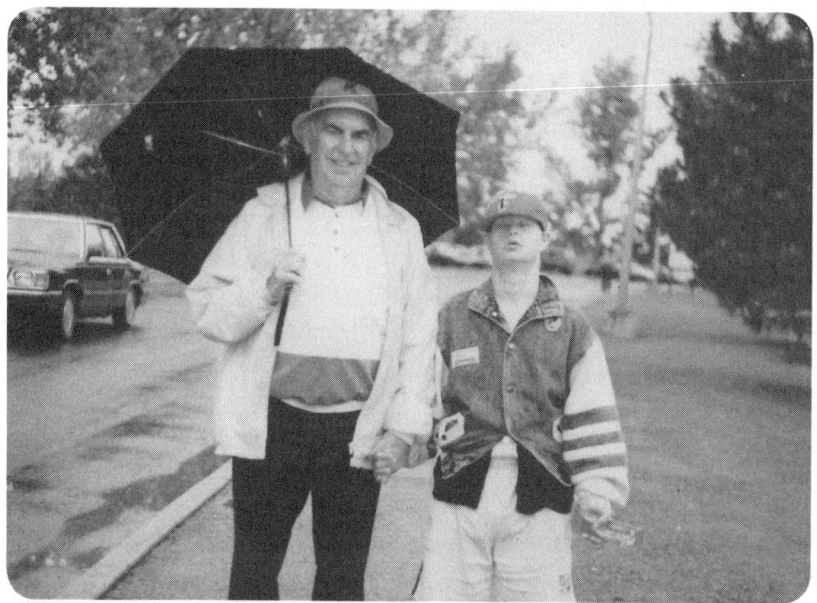

Family visits were always one way: we went to Smiths Falls to see Bill rather than having Bill come to Ottawa to see us. The Hershey chocolate factory—now closed—was a favourite stop on family visits.

Bill needed to perform rituals to ease his anxieties, at least temporarily. The more he was pushed to do something that interrupted his rituals or broke his need for order, the more anxious he became.

Anxiety disorders are the most common mental health problem in North America, including among people with Down syndrome.[7] OCD might explain a lot of things about Bill. But if he did have it, then a set of behaviours everyone else dismissed as harmless though sometimes annoying quirks—"just Bill being Bill," as one of his counsellors put it—may well have been signs of deep suffering. The fact it took until he was in his mid-thirties for anyone to figure this out is heartbreaking.

—

It was pretty clear by the time Bill was an adult that he was not the most likely candidate to flourish on the outside. He did have something many other residents at Smiths Falls lacked, however: he had a family who cared

about him, and visited him regularly. Bill's family—my family—lived in
a city with a number of group homes, possible family home placements,
and an active local association for people with disabilities. Our family
was also well off enough to give Bill whatever extra help he might have
needed. If my parents had pushed for him to move to Ottawa, that might
have made a difference.

They did not. And it's hard to understand why they opposed the idea.

Surely it would have been easier for Mom, with or without Dad, to
drive a few blocks to see Bill than to make the trek to Smiths Falls,
especially after her own health began to decline. If Bill lived in Ottawa,
she would have been able to see him more often, make sure he was doing
well, spoil him and his housemates now and then with little treats, and
maybe even include him in family events. Of course, group homes come
with their own problems,[8] but Mom and Dad could have been in the
background to keep an eye on things. They could have been articulate,
knowledgeable advocates on his behalf. I could have helped, too,
especially after I moved back to Ottawa in 1987. But I can't recall a single
family discussion about Bill moving to a home in Ottawa.

Mom made her views public in a rare letter to the editor of the *Ottawa
Citizen* in 1992, while the institution was launched on the long, slow
process of shutting down. She had been touched by a sentimental photo
essay about the adult residents at the institution, people for whom the
Rideau Regional Centre was the closest thing they had to a home. Here
is her letter, in full:

> I commend reporter Wanita Bates for her sensitive May
> 23 photo-story on Rideau Regional Centre in Smiths
> Falls. Too often in the past, the *Citizen* has concentrated
> only on the negative aspects of the facility. As parents of
> a long-time resident of Rideau Regional, we have been
> impressed and grateful for the care given to our son. The
> projected closing of the centre and the integration into

the community of the residents seem senseless — they
are already in a community where they are protected and
lovingly cared for.

Strange as it may sound, by the time she wrote the letter, she was
more or less right.

—

Bill's life inside the institution began changing for the better in the 1980s,
when he moved first to an independent living unit and then to a unit
known as Dundas, in the former nurses' residence. "Since our move to
Dundas on May 25, 1982, Billy has been a much happier young man,"
one of his counsellors wrote to my parents. "He is presently sharing a
room...and is much happier and much more contented." By this time the
restrictions on family visits to the living areas were long gone, and Mom
described his room to us. "Bill's room is like a jail cell, by choice, because
he resists all efforts to make it more attractive," she wrote. "Pictures I put

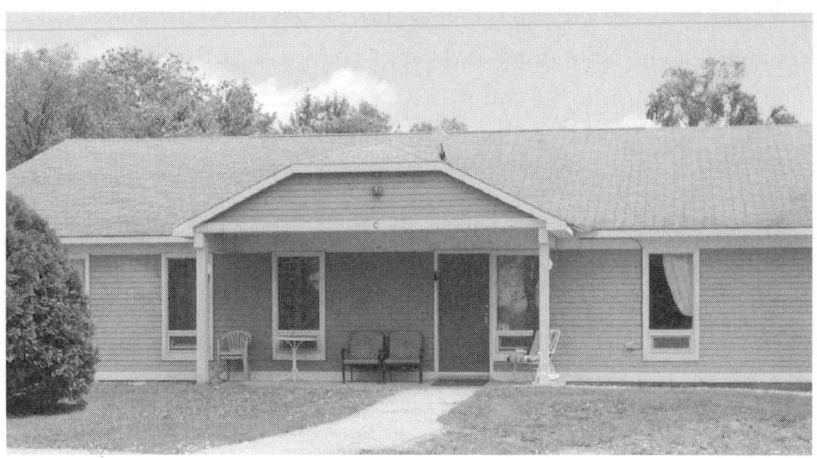

Modest though it was on the outside, Transition House C was Bill's happiest
home. It was one of a trio of bungalows on the institution grounds that
operated as a group home.

up were taken down, a table lamp was banished — even a radio I bought him was not wanted. When I insisted, he just took it to pieces after I left." Apparently, the habits of spartan living learned on the wards still held. Bill liked Dundas and was happy there, but the best years of his life began in the spring of 1990 when he moved into Transition House C, one of three grey bungalows on the grounds a short distance from the main building. Transition House C looked, felt, and operated like a family home, with a living room, dining room, kitchen, and a handful of bedrooms. As the name implied, it was meant to help residents get ready to move out of the institution and into the community.

Bill's counsellor reported to my parents that my brother was nervous about the move, but settled in quickly. The difference between this unit and the warehouse-style dorms he lived in as a child reflected the seismic shifts in policy and public attitudes that had occurred over the previous few decades. By 1990, Rideau Regional's population was less than a third of what it had been twenty years before, and the numbers were continuing to fall. The residents that remained were all adults. On the inside, the original idea behind the normalization movement — making the living arrangements look and feel more like real homes than institutions — had taken hold. The big wards were broken up into family-style apartments. The soulless dormitories and massive day rooms were pretty well gone. At Transition House C, Bill shared a room with another man with Down syndrome. Each had his own dresser and closet, which meant they had space to store private possessions (and, apparently, to hide food — another of Bill's quirks that showed up from time to time). He could go to his room when he felt like it, make himself a peanut butter sandwich in the kitchen, or go for a walk. The rigid barriers between the sexes had also fallen. Men and women spent time together, and some wards were mixed. Bill had a girlfriend, a cute and chatty redhead. The staff no longer wore uniforms that marked them as authority figures. Their job title was counsellor rather than ward aide, and they were much better trained. Vastly improved staff–resident ratios meant staff now had more time to get to know the residents, and to work with them one-on-one.

The invisible walls that kept the residents apart from the rest of the world were also gone. Bill, with the help of a counsellor, was able to go shopping in Smiths Falls or to the local Burger King or McDonald's. He and his fellow residents took bus trips to Niagara Falls, went to hockey games in Toronto, and took river cruises in Ottawa. He went to dances and parades and softball matches in communities surrounding Smiths Falls. Every summer he went to Grippen Lake Camp, used by Rideau Regional and many agencies from eastern Ontario and upper New York State. "Bill was up for anything," said Andy Shanks, who directed the camp. Bill loved to dance and watch the fireworks, and he took part in every theme day.[9] "He especially loved tubing behind the pontoon boat," Shanks recalled. "You could hear him laughing across the lake and calling for more." For a couple of years, he took courses in adaptive functioning at Algonquin College in Ottawa, taking a bus there and back five days a week.

At the institution, Bill walked by himself to work at the wood shop. Everybody he saw on the way knew him. He started working there in the early 1980s with a shift of one and half hours a day, which was upped to three hours a day and eventually to a full day. Bill wasn't paid for the work, but received an "incentive allowance" of six cents an hour, raised to nineteen cents in 1987.

He was also expected to take care of his room and do chores around the house. In this, he turned out to be a bit of a comedian—and what his Scottish ancestors would call a skiver. One of Bill's chores was to set the table for dinner. He did it badly. He dawdled and dragged his feet and fooled around and teased the counsellor supervising him, emoting like a diva in a melodrama and waiting for prompts to get back to the task at hand. The monthly reports from his counsellors on his progress in mastering this task are quite funny: "As always Bill can perform the task with much prompting from us and much grimacing on his part"; "Bill is up to the job if we are up to prodding"; "He doth protest too much but can perform the task up to house standards"; "Unfortunately still needs to be prompted constantly or supper will turn into breakfast. He would take that long"; and "Close supervision still required unless the others don't mind waiting an extra six hours for their meal."

He did no better with another chore, which was vacuuming his room on the weekend. He tended to choose one spot and go over it again and again—though whether this was a symptom of obsessive-compulsive disorder or sheer laziness is impossible to tell. As these counsellors' reports from 1991-92 show, it took an extraordinary amount of patience and prompting to get him to do the work completely:

> October: "Billy does a very good job at vacuuming. He needs help to start the vacuum and some prompts on directing but complies well. Seems to like the job!"

> November: "Vacuums relatively well once assisted with starting vacuum. Requires direction but sometimes can go ahead on his own but is waiting for prompts."

> January: "Still requires many prompts."

> February: "Can perform the task but supervision must be present."

> March: "Supervision and patience required to help see the task through."

> April: "Much prompting required."

> May: "Prompting required but can do the job independently."

> June: "Must be reminded to vacuum as he will not take it upon himself to do it. He does a good job but has to be verbally prompted along the way."

July: "No further progress. He will not do the task on his own initiative but certainly can do a fine job if he is constantly monitored."

August: "Although it required the usual amount of prompting Bill did a fine job whenever asked."

September: "As with the goal of setting the table Bill can be quite adept at vacuuming albeit with much guidance and finger pointing at untouched areas."

In the wood shop, Bill was part of a team that made duck decoys for sale outside the institution. His job was to sand the ducks, and it took him some time to adjust. According to an early vocational rehabilitation report, in 1981, "His overall work performance to date has been marginal. . . . He requires close supervision and, at times, his behaviour can be disruptive. It is very difficult to keep him on task and, if not closely watched, [he] will bother the other workers." But, as he became more and more comfortable in the wood shop, he grew to enjoy it. Andy Shanks, who got to know Bill's work when he took over the shop a few years later, said Bill was a good worker. He took pride in what he did and liked to get praise for doing a good job. But no one could accuse him of being a rate buster. One of his counsellors told us he was the kind of guy who showed up for work late, went for coffee break early, and did his best to stretch the coffee break until quitting time. But he was fun to be around, and everyone in the shop knew him and was happy to see him arrive. "Work was all about the camaraderie," Shanks said. "He was always in the middle of every practical joke. He loved to laugh with you, not at you. That was one of the things we loved about Bill." At the end of each shift he saluted, said "la" (probably short for "later") to Shanks and the people in the work area, and headed out the door with a hint of a swagger.

One thing Bill really liked to work on was what the rest of us called colouring, but what he may have seen as art. His medium was crayons on colouring book, and his preferred working space was in front of the television. He was fastidious about his crayons, peeling the paper to the right level and rejecting any that broke. When he was in the mood to create, he chose a fresh page in whatever colouring book he had on hand and started to work. Though he could colour within the lines, according to a 1979 report, he preferred a more free-form approach. He ignored the lines completely, drawing great loops and scrawls of colour. Mom, who painted lovely and carefully composed acrylic landscapes, once joked that he was a budding abstract expressionist. Sometimes he would stop a project and snort in disgust, apparently over a mistake he had made. The fact no one else could see the mistake didn't matter; he could, and once a picture was ruined, he wouldn't touch it again. No one else could tell when a picture was complete either, but Bill could. When he was done, he was done. For his next work, he needed a fresh page in the colouring book. He didn't hang up his pictures, and I'm not sure he ever looked at them again once he was finished — simply making them was good enough.

"Bill was a happy and jovial guy," recalls Sandy Baker Lennox, his primary counsellor at Transition House C in 1990-91. "Coming from a care provider, he had a wonderful life."[10]

The psychologist who thought Bill should try a medication used to treat obsessive-compulsive disorder probably saw his behaviour at work and play — including the constant need for prompts — as symptoms of the condition, and he was probably right, at least in part. But I think there was another side to Bill's behaviour. By the time he was in his thirties, Bill had figured out a couple of the secrets of institutional life. One was that whether he set the table properly or folded his clothes the right way, or sanded two ducks instead of one or vacuumed the whole rug rather than one patch, really didn't matter all that much. He was still going to eat, he was still going to have his bed to sleep in, and no one would fire him or cast him out. He knew that if he really misbehaved he would lose privileges, like going to the institution's coffee house, so he rarely misbehaved aggressively. He liked getting attention from the staff, so he figured out how to do this without pushing them (or himself) too far. He loved to laugh and play jokes on people. He teased and fooled around, slowed his typically molasses-like pace to glacier speed when he objected to what was going on, and controlled whatever scraps of his life he could control. He took out many of his anxieties in private, pulling out an eyebrow or checking his food stash or stuffing a rag in his shoe or his underpants, or peeling his crayons until they were just so. When he was with other people and felt sad or uncomfortable, he displayed his misery flamboyantly in hopes someone would make him feel better. When someone came to his aid, his smile shone with delight.

At least one of his counsellors interpreted his over-the-top behaviour as a con job, and that may have been partly right, too. But I remember that grin of his—it could melt hearts.

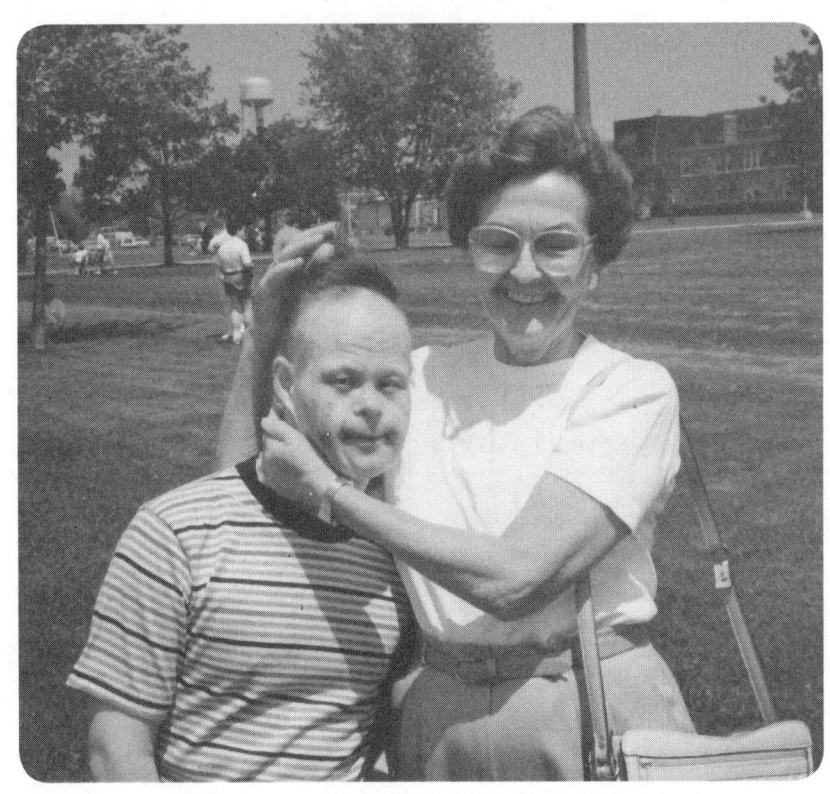

When I reconnected with Bill after several years away, I was shocked at how
old he looked. In this photo taken at Rideau Regional's family day in 1989,
he was 32 and had been a resident of the institution for 30 years.

Chapter 9

"INCLUSION, INDEPENDENCE AND CHOICE"

By the middle of the 1970s, pretty well anyone with a stake in the big residential Ontario institutions for people with intellectual disabilities thought the end was near.

Walter Williston's far-ranging 1971 report, which called for a phase-out of the institutions as quickly as possible, had energized the proponents of community care. Two years later, the influential provincial cabinet minister Robert Welch had committed Ontario to the idea that "wherever feasible, services should be provided in a community setting as an alternative to institutionalization." The principles behind the normalization movement had become—well, normalized. Jean Vanier's growing L'Arche movement—founded in France in 1964, it opened its first house in Canada five years later—was showing how people with intellectual disabilities could be full-fledged participants in their communities instead of patients. All signs pointed in the same direction: people with intellectual disabilities did not need to be shut away in hospital schools. With the right help and support, they could thrive outside the institutions. They could go to school, find jobs, have romances, take part in social, political, and cultural activities, and become valued and valuable members of their community. In taking this stance, Ontario had become a world leader, one of the first jurisdictions anywhere to incorporate the principles of normalization and community living into social policy.[1]

But anyone who thought the doors to those institutions were about to close was in for a shock. It did not happen in five years, or ten, or even twenty. The oldest and biggest institutions, Huronia at Orillia and Rideau Regional in Smiths Falls, stayed in business until the spring of 2009, a stunning thirty-eight years after Williston's report. Williston was long dead by then. So was Welch. Pierre Berton, whose 1960 *Toronto Star* column on Huronia energized critics of the institutional approach, would not live to see the lights go off for the last time. Nor would my brother Bill.

So what took so long?

The simple answer is that there is no simple answer. A whole lot of issues and realities got in the way: slow-moving bureaucracies, opposition from expected and unexpected sources, tight-fisted governments, shifts in political power, twists and turns in policy that created new uncertainties even as they solved old problems. The needs of people like my brother rarely made it to the top of the political agenda. When they did, it tended to be at moments of crisis or opportunity, moments that would energize a government for a while and then fade away. There are few villains in this story, and fewer heroes. In the end, Ontario did the right thing and acknowledged that the institutions had been a failure. But it took a long, long time to reach that end.

The starting point for shutting down the institutional system came in 1973, when the government decided to shift responsibility for the institutions from the health ministry to the community and social services ministry. A critical piece of legislation passed that year, the Developmental Services Act, put an end to decades of policy-making that equated intellectual disabilities with illnesses requiring hospital-based treatment and, in many cases, treatment for life. Hard though it is to imagine today, by the time this legislation passed, my basically healthy teenaged brother had been officially classed as a hospital patient for almost sixteen of his eighteen years. The new act established community living as the preferred choice for people like Bill, and provided funding for community-based services such as group homes, family homes with support services, day programs, sheltered workshops, and skills training programs. It also acknowledged the need to provide help and support to the tens of thousands of families that had kept children with disabilities at home. The goal of the act was both noble and ambitious: overcoming the physical, economic, and social conditions that kept people with disabilities from full inclusion in society.

Simply assessing the extent of the problem that needed to be solved by the act was harder than it might seem, however. The number of people living in institutions owned and operated by the government—known as Schedule 1 institutions—peaked in 1974 at roughly eight thousand.[2] A 1973 consultants' report counted another 2,350 people with intellectual disabilities in the Homes for Special Care, which had been established in the 1960s. About two thousand more were in psychiatric institutions, fourteen hundred in nursing homes, and 450 in a kind of foster home. About four hundred children were living in eleven nursing homes specifically for children with intellectual disabilities.[3]

Transferring the Schedule 1 institutions—the big Huronia, Rideau, and Southwestern Ontario facilities, plus roughly a dozen smaller centres[4]—to the community and social services ministry gave the province access to money from the Canada Assistance Plan. But almost as many people with intellectual disabilities remained in nursing homes or psychiatric hospitals, which were still under the health ministry. They continued to be seen as patients: people who needed medical care, rather than social assistance. As a result, federal money wasn't available for them.

Regardless of which ministry was in charge, the level of care individuals in the provincial system needed varied widely. Some were completely bedridden, unable to chew or swallow food. Others had a combination of physical, psychological, and intellectual disabilities. Some had chronic medical conditions, with or without an intellectual disability. This group included Justin Clark, who was sent to Rideau Regional at the age of two because he had cerebral palsy and could not walk or talk. When he became an adult, Clark took his parents to court and proved he was mentally competent to make his own life decisions. The case is viewed as a milestone in the fight for disability rights.[5] Many, like my brother, were able to eat, use the toilet, and dress by themselves but were unable to speak, read, count, or handle money. Some had little or no developmental deficits but had been hard to place in foster care as children, and wound up in the institutions more or less by default. If community care was the goal, it should be the goal for all. Given the diversity of the population, however, there was no one-size-fits-all solution.

Williston had noted in his 1971 report that, regardless of the level of the intellectual disability, long-term residents of institutions suffered social deficits. Institutional life, he argued, forced people to function far below their developmental capabilities. Because their lives had been so regimented and controlled, they would have to learn from scratch how to make the simplest decisions about life on the outside. They would also be stigmatized as former institution residents, and overcoming these deficits would be neither simple nor quick.

York University political scientist Harvey G. Simmons writes that the policy shift toward community care triggered "a period of conflict, confusion and uncertainty" inside the community and social services ministry as the people in charge of restructuring the system disagreed over how to do it.[6] Some argued for breaking the big institutions up into smaller ones; others rejected pretty well every aspect of the institutional model.

And then there was the problem of public perception. When the move to community care started in the early 1970s, politicians talked about a 50 or 60 per cent cut in the institutional population within five years. By the spring of 1976, in the wake of some violent incidents at Huronia, Community and Social Services Minister James Taylor fretted about a possible backlash if the province moved too quickly in returning institution residents to their communities. "We have to educate the community," Taylor told the annual conference of the Ontario Association for the Mentally Retarded. "It's a two-way street and don't think I don't struggle with that in the Orillia area."[7] Ontario residents generally favoured normalization in theory, but many saw people with disabilities as strange, scary, and possibly dangerous — in other words, as undesirable neighbours. Some worried that group homes would disrupt their neigbourhoods and reduce property values. The Metropolitan Toronto Association for the Mentally Retarded ran into zoning problems in every part of Toronto where it planned to open group homes. "Everyone is in favour of group homes, only 'not on my street,'" the association's president, James Turner, told the *Globe and Mail* in 1976. In the Toronto suburb of Etobicoke, for example, the association had rented an ideal house, but it was sitting empty because of a zoning dispute.[8] Other associations ran into the same problem, and have continued to do so for decades. A 2012 article in *Canadian Lawyer* noted that complaints about municipal zoning bylaws discriminating against disabled people and other vulnerable groups had become increasingly common.[9] In 2014 Toronto city councillor Doug Ford — now Ontario's premier — complained that a group home for three to five youth with developmental disabilities had "ruined" a neighbourhood in his ward. The neighbours of the home, worried about home values and potential damage to property, applauded his comments.[10] Others did not. "I asked my wife, is it 2014 or 1914?" said Chris Beesley, head of Community Living Ontario. "This seems to be such a step backwards."[11]

Deinstitutionalization also revived an ugly idea from the eugenics era: involuntary sterilization of people with intellectual disabilities. In 1973, an employee of the Metropolitan Toronto Association for the Mentally Retarded proposed that compulsory sterilization should be a condition for acceptance into any group home subsidized by the province. The association's director of residences, who opposed the idea, resigned over the issue. In a memo to another member of the legislature, the provincial secretary for social development, Robert Welch, wrote: "We must certainly not allow this policy to become established by default rather than a conscious examination of all the alternatives."[12]

The sterilization issue came up in the Ontario legislature several times during the 1970s. In 1978, the health minister was asked about a study that found 686 people who were unable to give consent were sterilized in general hospitals across Ontario in 1976. Some 308 were children, all but fifty of them girls. Ontario's public guardian argued that the sterilizations of adults were probably illegal because the individuals were unable to give consent.[13] Parents could give consent for surgery on children under sixteen, and it appears many opted for surgery before their children hit that age, or at the first sign of sexual maturity. Aides to the minister of community and social services put together briefing notes that counted sixty-five sterilization operations on institution residents between 1970 and 1976, and another forty-four in 1977 and 1978.[14] In Quebec, more than five hundred people with intellectual disabilities, many of them children, were sterilized between 1976 and 1978.[15] The rush to the surgical option, with all its attendant risks, is astounding. A Supreme Court of Canada decision outlawed involuntary sterilization of people with intellectual disabilities in the 1980s.

An even more shocking study made public in the late 1970s found that some families and doctors had denied life-saving surgery to infants with Down syndrome. The Canadian Psychiatric Association said a twenty-year study at the Hospital for Sick Children in Toronto had found that twenty-seven of fifty children with Down syndrome and a blocked food passage in the stomach were allowed to die from an "easily correctable lesion" that prevented them from swallowing food. "This increasingly common act in medical practice is being vigorously promoted by able and influential advocates within our profession and within our society at large," the association's statement said. A Montreal doctor began advocating that doctors withhold treatment from children with Down syndrome in 1974, the association's statement added, and the practice had gained support ever since. "These are not times in which we should be either starting or expanding the practice of letting mongoloid infants die."[16]

While the government wrestled with how—and under what circumstances—to get people back out into the community, and with how to get the community to accept them, it faced internal debate about the meaning of normalization. Some officials in the Ministry of Community and Social Services argued that normalization could go on inside the institutions by redesigning wards into family-style units with no more than ten people per unit, and by rethinking how residents might make better use of their time for work, school, and leisure. Others in the public service argued that normalization and institutionalization were polar opposites. People with intellectual disabilities needed individually tailored supports that would allow them to become fully participating citizens of their communities, they contended, not prettier institutions. These advocates of community care believed that the ministry should, in essence, cut its losses on the institutions and devote all resources to the community development program.[17] Ultimately the province ended up pursuing both ideas, and more besides. By 1977 it had opened three new 150-bed institutions and was planning a fourth. It was pushing ahead with plans to cut the populations of Huronia, Rideau, and Southwestern Ontario quickly and deeply, in part through transfers to these new centres. And it was pursuing plans to move people into a wide variety of community homes.

The province was also beginning to deal with problems arising from some of its earlier efforts at getting people out of the big institutions. The most troublesome was the Homes for Special Care program. These privately owned and publicly funded nursing homes had been established in the 1960s for former psychiatric patients, but soon opened their doors to people with intellectual disabilities. By the early 1970s, approximately twenty-three hundred people with intellectual disabilities were living in these homes, hundreds more than in Huronia itself.[18]

In many ways, the province's seemingly well-intentioned effort to get people out of the big institutions created living situations that were throwbacks to the darker days of institutional care. While the residences provided food and shelter to their residents, they were not required to offer recreation, exercise, therapy, or activities. The people running the homes, known as hosts and hostesses, needed no specialized training, or any level of formal education. A series of media reports and studies in the 1970s found that many of the people living in homes associated with Homes for Special Care were worse off than they had been in an institution. A 1976 *Globe and Mail* article, for example, described lives of tedium and isolation.[19] Residents spent their days watching TV or waiting for the next meal. There was nothing else for them to do. In one home, reporter Rosemarie Boyle wrote, "eighteen profoundly retarded young adults lie together on mats or slump in wheelchairs in a sparse playroom because their activity person is away that day." In another, "forty-five men and women spend their days sitting in a large room with little to look forward to but the next meal, a cigarette, or their daily chores." One-third of the homes housed a dozen or more people, which meant they bore little or no resemblance to family homes. The health ministry employees assigned to monitor the homes, meanwhile, carried enormous caseloads of 265 residents each.[20] With that many individuals to monitor, it was impossible for employees to do anything other than ensure a resident had enough to eat and a place to sleep.

Worst of all, 325 children were living in these homes.[21] The vast majority of these children received nothing but nursing care; only twenty had any kind of educational program set up for them, and what they had was meagre. The Ontario Association for the Mentally Retarded, which had been campaigning for years to get Homes for Special Care transferred from the health ministry to the same ministry that ran the big institutions, seized on this issue. The health ministry spent the equivalent of $28 per day to take care of each resident, while community and social services spent $51 a day for residents in its care—a disparity that raised accusations that the government was saving money on the backs of those least able to defend their own interests.[22] Eventually, the province stepped in with reforms, but only after years of pressure and after a series of negative media reports.

Despite all the difficulties the province faced in reorienting the system toward community care, it made progress. Many of those early moves turned out to be quite successful, as in the case of Beverly Scullion's sister, Gayle St. George. Born in 1953 with Down syndrome and admitted to the Rideau Regional Centre when she was two and a half, Gayle moved to a group home in Renfrew in the early 1970s. "When my parents were first approached about the move, they were not keen," Scullion recalls. "Fear of the unknown, I guess." After talking to other parents and people at the institution, they agreed to the move. Gayle did well. She lived in a bungalow, where she had her own room. She went to work down the road at a sheltered workshop. The house became her home; she and her roommates shared shopping and kitchen duties, and family and friends could visit. She could have parties to celebrate birthdays or other occasions. She went to restaurants; she chose her own clothes. "She was a happy-go-lucky gal," her sister says. Gayle lived at the Renfrew group home until she died of heart failure at forty-one.[23]

Between 1975 and 1982, the community and social services ministry increased its annual budget for community services for developmentally handicapped people from $10 million to $118 million. The ministry also created twenty-eight hundred new community living places, and more than doubled the capacity of the workshop and employment training system. "The development of these and other resources allowed some thirty-eight hundred residents of institutions for the developmentally handicapped in Ontario to move back to the community, and it reduced the overall population of these institutions by fourteen hundred," minister Frank Drea told the Ontario legislature in 1983.[24] The number of residents at Smiths Falls had fallen to one thousand, Huronia's population stood at 967, and just 654 people were living at the Southwestern Regional Centre, Drea said. He reminded the legislature that the province was in the early months of a new five-year plan for getting more people out of the institutions and back into the community. This plan, announced the previous October, would create hundreds of group homes. It would also provide money for family support and job training, create jobs for nineteen hundred adults, and set up new beds for severely handicapped children and adults.

The most radical part of the ministry's plan was closing six institutions. All were among the smaller institutions, and they were located all over the province. At the time Drea gave his update, the St. Lawrence

Centre in Brockville was two months away from closing, and the
Bluewater Centre in Goderich, near Lake Huron, was next on the list.
The details on where those residents went offer insights into both the
achievements and difficulties of the move.

Drea reported, in his 1983 speech, that fifty-five St. Lawrence residents
had already moved out of the institution, and that plans were in place
for the remaining forty-five. Those who left had, truly, been scattered all
over the province. Twenty had moved to existing community residences
in eight different communities; nine were living with a host family in the
family home program in four different towns; twenty moved to one or
another of the provincial institutions; and three were in the Brockville
psychiatric hospital. Only three had moved back to their hometowns.
"When the institution closes, seventy-four of the one hundred residents
will be living in group homes and family homes in the community, and
another six residents will be ready to move back to the community within
two to three years, after they receive the additional training they require,"
Drea said. "This means our earlier prediction regarding the number of
residents who would be capable of community living was overcautious.
The great majority will now enjoy a fuller life outside an institution.
This shows what can be achieved when carefully planned community
alternatives are provided."[25]

Six months later, acting minister Bruce McCaffrey — filling in
for an ailing Drea — told the legislature that eight of the seventy-five
St. Lawrence residents who had moved to community living arrangements
were back in institutional care, most of them at the Rideau Regional
Centre. McCaffrey also reported that sixty-seven of the one hundred
fifty Bluewater Centre residents had been moved, forty-two of them to
community residences and twenty-five to other institutions. Another
forty were due for transfer to another institution, almost all of them
going to the Midwestern Regional Centre in Palmerston. McCaffrey
said the moves from one institution to the other came about because of
"program needs, parental requests, or to bring these individuals closer to
their homes."[26]

By starting with the smaller facilities, the province hoped to eat away at the institutional system from the edges, moving people who were most likely to adapt to the community into group homes, family homes, or other community living arrangements, and transferring people whose disabilities were more challenging to other institutions. At the same time, all over Ontario, the families of the residents of those smaller institutions were fearful and anxious, unsure when or where the resident would be moved. The residents were worried too: change was in the air, but all they knew was that they would probably be separated from the people they knew best. Some worried that, having left Huronia or Rideau Regional for one of the smaller institutions just a few years earlier, they might end up back where they started when the smaller institution closed. In short, many families, residents, and people who worked with people with disabilities feared that what was really going on was a giant game of musical chairs.

By the end of its five-year plan, the province closed four institutions, not six. And then suddenly, in 1985, all plans were up in the air.

—

No political party had more impact on the intellectually disabled in Canada than Ontario's Conservatives. The party was in power for all but five years between 1905 and 1934, the years when the Orillia Asylum for Idiots grew into the mammoth Ontario Hospital School and when Smiths Falls was chosen as the site for a second large institution. The Conservatives returned to power in 1943, and stayed there for the next forty-two years. During these decades Conservative governments oversaw the construction, expansion, and rehabilitation of all the other residential institutions for people with intellectual disabilities. Conservative governments made the laws on education, first keeping children with severe disabilities out of school, then providing limited classes and special schools, then permitting integration in the regular public schools, and ultimately enacting a law that guaranteed special education programs and special education services for children in their home communities.

Conservative governments made ground-breaking policy decisions promoting community care. But by the mid-1980s, for reasons that had nothing to do with disability policy, Ontario voters were ready for a change. The May 1985 election ended in a stalemate: the Conservatives won fifty-two seats, the Liberals forty-eight, and the New Democrats twenty-five. The Liberals, with the support of the New Democrats, took control. The Liberals turned their minority government into a majority in an election two years later.

Though people like my brother Bill had nothing to do with these shifts in power, their lives would nonetheless be affected.

The Liberal government released its own plan for people with developmental disabilities in May of 1987. Titled *Challenges and Opportunities*, it set out basically the same long-term goals as those of the previous Conservative governments: phasing out the institutions and establishing a comprehensive system of services that would allow people with intellectual handicaps to stay in their home communities.[27] Long term, in this case, meant about twenty-five years. The Liberal plan also addressed a simmering short-term problem that was threatening to come to a boil. By clamping down on admissions to the institutions and concentrating on getting existing residents out, the province had paid too little attention to people with disabilities who had never lived in an institution. These people were already in the community and they needed care, including housing, employment, and other supports.

Challenges and Opportunities estimated that about seventy-eight thousand Ontario residents had developmental handicaps, and at any one time forty-four thousand of them would need training and support. But in 1987, only thirty-three thousand people—eight thousand in institutions and nursing homes and twenty-five thousand in the community—had access to the help they needed.[28] The Liberal government promised that it would respond to what it called "pent-up demand" for services from people living in the community, in nursing homes, and in institutions. Over the next seven years, this would include residential, supported-living, employment, and day program services for up to nine thousand of these people. It would also provide new community living arrangements for one thousand institution residents, and for another thousand people who were staying in nursing homes. Any children still living in nursing homes at that point would be moved to better living arrangements within a year.

This government didn't have seven years to carry out its short-term plan. A snap election the Liberals called in 1990 turned out to be a disaster for the party. By October 1, the Liberals were out and the New Democratic Party was in. This government took power at the onset of a recession that hit Ontario particularly hard. Bob Rae's five years as premier were tumultuous: he drew fire from the right for refusing to back away from some core economic and social principles, and from the left for backtracking on election promises, freezing public sector pay, and forcing public sector workers to work without pay for twelve days a year. The New Democrats went through three community and social services ministers during their five years in office. The first, Zanana Akande, had to step aside over a conflict of interest; the second, Marion Boyd, held the job for fifteen months before being promoted to attorney general; and the third, Tony Silipo, mainly concentrated on shepherding a comprehensive welfare reform package through the legislature. Services for people with developmental handicaps did not fall off the table, but developing policy in the area was a relatively low priority. By the end of the Rae government's term in office, only two more of the smaller institutions had closed.

In 1995 the New Democrats were bounced out of power and into third-party status as the Conservatives returned to power under Mike Harris. These Conservatives, however, were nothing like the Conservatives that ran Ontario in the first four decades of the post-war era. While the old-time Conservatives did not always get things right, and could never be accused of erring on the side of generosity, they believed that governments had a political, social, and moral obligation to provide a social welfare system for the disadvantaged, including for people with intellectual disabilities.

Mike Harris's Conservatives took a radically different view, based on the idea that government itself was the biggest problem facing Ontario and that bureaucracy and taxes were suppressing social and economic development. Harris promised deep tax cuts, widespread privatization of government services, smaller bureaucracies, and balanced budgets.[29] Almost immediately after taking office, the government announced cuts of 22 per cent in social assistance rates. It argued that people were taking advantage of welfare, and that government assistance was a disincentive to finding work. The welfare issue was so fraught and controversial that the point man on the policy, community and social services minister David Tsubouchi, had little time for anything else in his year in that portfolio. Cuts in other areas followed. By the late 1990s, the Harris Conservatives had cut deeply into health, education, and community programs; reduced the number of school boards in the province to seventy-two from 129; begun forced amalgamations of municipalities; implemented workfare; and frozen the minimum wage.[30]

Advocates for people with disabilities, accustomed under previous governments to lobbying for more and better support, found themselves on the losing end of a struggle to keep what they had. After a wholesale review of its social services policies, the government proposed privatizing some programs for people with intellectual disabilities, deregulating others, and imposing user fees for services that until then had come free of charge.[31] The Ottawa-Carleton Association for Persons with Developmental Disabilities calls the two terms of this government "The Harris Hell."

"Harris's main act in disabilities was 'Making Services Work for People' which, if you talk to most parents at the time, was the exact opposite of what it did," the association's website says. The Harris government's policy was based on streamlining and rationalizing services, and on moving away from government-provided services to what it called "shared responsibility" — basically, shifting more of the burden of care to families and communities. "The legislation was made without consultation of the public involved with developmental disability services, and for an active group rooted in parent activism, this did not sit well," the association notes. "The cuts proposed weren't going to cover the services needed and would leave an already vulnerable population even more at risk."[32]

It's fair to say that none of the four people who served as community and social services ministers from the time of the Conservatives' initial victory in 1995 to their defeat in 2003 saw services for people with intellectual disabilities as their top priority. Other issues, especially their multi-pronged efforts to cut the welfare rolls and reduce spending, occupied their attention. The Conservatives did close the remaining smaller institutions between 1996 and 1999, however, and moved several hundred residents into the community. John Baird, who was minister in May 2000, announced a $50 million program to help people with disabilities integrate into the community.[33] He intimated later that year that the province was considering closing the last three institutions — Huronia, Rideau Regional, and Southwestern Ontario — but little happened to advance that idea.[34] When the Liberals took power in Ontario again in 2003, closing the institutions moved up on the political agenda.

—

Back in 1973, when Robert Welch's green paper promised a move to community care, "Ontario was ahead of its time," says Don Gallant, national director of the Ready, Willing and Able project, which works with employers to create inclusive work forces. "The time it took to complete that circle is another story."[35] Over the years that followed, other jurisdictions surpassed Ontario, with Newfoundland and Labrador and British Columbia leading the way. Newfoundland adopted a policy of deinstitutionalization in 1982 and closed its two state-run institutions for people with intellectual disabilities: the Children's Home in 1983 and Exon House in 1988.[36] British Columbia announced in 1981 that it would close its large Woodlands institution, which had opened in the late nineteenth century and, by the 1950s, housed roughly fourteen hundred people. It shut down in 1996. In response to allegations made by former residents, the province launched a review that found evidence of systemic abuse at Woodlands, including physical, sexual, and emotional abuse. Residents had been beaten, kicked, shackled, isolated, bullied, and sexually assaulted. A class-action suit on behalf of former residents, settled in 2010, offered them compensation ranging from $3,000 to $150,000 depending on the severity of the abuse. Another group of former Woodlands residents, who had been shut out of the initial settlement because of a legal technicality, received compensation in 2018.[37]

Other provinces have closed their institutions too. By 2018, Gallant says, only three government-funded institutions operated specifically for people with intellectual disabilities remained: the Michener Centre in Alberta, the Manitoba Developmental Centre, and Valley View in Saskatchewan. Gallant estimates that together they held roughly six hundred residents. Saskatchewan has announced that Valley View will close and has been moving residents out. Alberta announced and then rescinded plans to close the Michener Centre, following complaints that the closing would cause chaos for vulnerable people. The Manitoba Developmental Centre in Portage la Prairie continues to operate, housing about a hundred people at the time of writing. The Centre, which opened in 1890, once had twelve hundred residents. Former residents of Valley View and the Manitoba Developmental Centre have filed class action suits alleging physical, psychological, and sexual abuse.[38]

Other countries have also been shutting down their own institutional systems. In England, the population in institutions dropped from fifty-one thousand in 1976 to less than four thousand in 2002, while Australia has experienced a similar trend. Sweden and Norway have closed all their institutions. In the United States, 115 institutions closed between the 1960s and the 1990s, and the institutionalized population dropped 70 per cent: from 194,650 in 1967 to 48,496 in 1999.[39]

Some of the best-known—or most notorious—institutions were gone long before Ontario's. Willowbrook on New York City's Staten Island, at one time the biggest institution of its kind in the United States and plagued by scandal, closed in 1987. Letchworth Village, once touted as the model "village of the simple," shut down in 1996.[40] The most famous institution of them all, John Langdon Down's Normansfield Hospital in London, shut down the following year. The fear of the feeble-minded that characterized the early years of the twentieth century had had an impact on Normansfield. Though it looked much the same as ever from the outside, it became a custodial institution, like the big public institutions in North America. Normansfield fell on hard times in the 1970s. Dr. Terence Lawlor, who had taken over in 1971 after the retirement of Down's grandson Norman, alienated his medical and nursing staff, who felt he was both arrogant and incompetent. Conditions inside the hospital deteriorated and, in May of 1976, most of the nursing staff went on strike to demand Lawlor's suspension, leaving the residents alone inside. The walkout was a scandal and prompted a lengthy inquiry, after which Lawlor and a number of nursing administrators were fired. A decision to close the hospital was made in the 1980s, and it finally shut down in 1997.[41]

Ontario's institutions closed without scandals of the sort seen elsewhere, but not without controversy — or opposition. It turned out that, after years of slow deinstitutionalization, a number of groups — provincial and municipal politicians, local businesses, the public service employees union, and many parents like my own — did not want to see the institutions shut down at all. Sandra Pupatello, the community and social services minister in the new Liberal government, announced in the fall of 2004 that the final three institutions would close by the end of March 2009. Before that date, the province would spend $110 million on community services for the remaining one thousand residents. About $70 million of this was to go toward new housing, some of it with twenty-four-hour care. "We will complete a long-standing journey from an institution-based service system for people with developmental disabilities to a community-based system that promotes inclusion, independence and choice," Pupatello said. Disability advocates, like Michael Bach of the Canadian Association for Community Living, welcomed the announcement. "For

Ontario, with the largest number of people institutionalized, to make the financial and political commitment to do this bodes well for finishing the job of closing institutions in this country," he told the *Globe and Mail*.[42]

But if getting people out of the institutions in the 1970s and 1980s had been difficult, the job was even harder now.

The big institutions traditionally housed a mix of children and adults. In 1972, for example, roughly one-quarter of the residents were children under fourteen and one-fifth were teens aged fifteen to eighteen. People over forty accounted for about 10 per cent of the total population. The rest were young adults. By 2003, after years of limited admissions and steady efforts to move people into the community, the average age of a resident was forty-nine. The youngest were in their twenties, the oldest in their nineties. Many, including people in their forties and fifties, had age-related conditions like osteoporosis or Alzheimer's disease on top of their other disabilities. Ninety per cent of them had lived in an institution for twenty years or more, and the average length of stay was thirty-eight years.[43] Many had little or no family—their parents, if they were still alive, were themselves elderly and frail—and no conception of daily life on the outside.

Norm Sterling, the Conservative MPP whose riding included Smiths Falls, told the Ontario legislature that it would be impossible to provide adequate care for the remaining residents anywhere other than the institution. "I'm calling on the minister to immediately reverse this decision. Let the remaining residents live out the rest of their lives with their life-long friends," he urged. "Don't separate them from the physical and emotional surroundings which they have relied on virtually all of their lives. I will continue to advocate for the well-being of these residents and ensure they don't fall through the cracks."[44]

The Ontario Public Service Employees Union, which represented the workers at the three institutions, called the decision "heartless" and "a tragic mistake," and urged the minister to reconsider. "These aren't just buildings; to the residents it's home," the union's president, Leah Casselman, said in a news release: "A lot of the residents of these centres have lived there all of their lives. These people cannot function in a community setting." The institutions, she argued, "are staffed by trained professionals who are quite simply the best in the province at caring for these residents." Both OPSEU and the politicians representing the communities where the institutions were located also warned that the closings would take an enormous economic toll on those communities. "The loss of these jobs is an economic earthquake to Orillia, Smiths Falls, and Blenheim," Casselman said. "This is a total of $84.4 million being taken out of Ontario's economy. We're talking about nearly two thousand jobs that will leave these communities and never return."[45]

Over the next few years Sterling, and other MPPs whose ridings contained the institutions, read into the public record a number of petitions to keep the centres open.[46] Some focused on the needs of the residents and their families. "Many of these elderly parents can't physically care for their adult children themselves, and they are afraid that the move from RRC [Rideau Regional Centre] will hurt their children both physically and emotionally," Sterling said as be brought forward one petition with sixty-five hundred signatures. Other petitions focused on the impact of the closing on the local economies. The situation in Smiths Falls was especially dire because the town's two biggest employers, Rideau Regional and the Hershey chocolate plant, were both shutting down. A petition Sterling read into the record in 2007 called for action on two fronts: getting Hershey to reverse its decision to move to Mexico, and postponing the closing of the Rideau Regional Centre until the province had created as many public sector jobs in the town as would be lost when the institution closed.

Families of Rideau Regional residents, joined by a group of families from Huronia, went to court to block the closings.[47] They argued that community homes could not match the facilities and services available in the institution. Rideau Regional had an infirmary, medical and dental clinics, physiotherapy facilities, and a range of programs offering comprehensive on-site medical, nursing, and psychiatric services. It also provided specialized services for residents with Alzheimer's disease, behavioural problems, or vision problems. Its recreational facilities ranged from a swimming pool to a bowling alley to a summer camp. The swimming pool had specialized equipment to help improve the prospects of people with osteoporosis, cerebral palsy, or the risk of muscular atrophy. All of this would be lost to residents if they had to leave the institution. The suit also argued that the government had no legal authority to close down the facilities, and that transferring residents without properly obtained informed consent would be a breach of their rights under the Canadian Charter of Rights and Freedoms.

The three-judge panel that heard the case released a unanimous decision in January 2006. It said the province did indeed have the right to shut down the facilities, but it also said that residents could not be transferred to group homes or other facilities without the consent of the individuals, their family, or their guardian. In the event of a disagreement, the province would have to apply to Superior Court to proceed. Disability advocates saw the ruling on consent as a victory. Lawyer Doug Elliott, speaking for the families of Huronia residents, said a number of unsuitable resident placements had been "foisted on families" over the years. That wouldn't happen any more, he added: "Families have the right to determine if a placement is in the best interest of the relative and if it's not suitable, they can say no and no means no."[48]

Over the next few years, the province pushed ahead with creating places in the community for the remaining 941 institution residents. The moves were anything but simple. Researchers with the Centre for Applied Disability Studies at Brock University, commissioned by the government to report on the transition, put together a set of case studies looking at individual residents moving out of Huronia, Rideau Regional, and Southwestern.[49] The studies show the remarkably complex requirements many of these people had, regardless of where they lived.

"Margaret," fifty-eight, had cataracts, hearing loss in both ears, curvature of the spine, a skin condition, a heart condition, osteoporosis, and epilepsy. Born with Down syndrome, she had lived in an institution since the age of five. She needed twenty-four-hour, seven-day-a-week care. "Peter," forty-seven, had a profound intellectual disability due to an unidentified genetic disorder and had lived in an institution from the age of five. He had a history of hurting himself, hurting others, and trying to run away. He flipped furniture, broke windows, charged at staff and peers, yelled, screamed, and threw objects. Once he punched through a glass window, severing an artery in his arm. Sometimes he masturbated in public. He had limited speech and did not interact with his roommates, going to the staff when he needed things. His ability to make decisions was impaired. "Angie," fifty-two, had a rare genetic neurological and developmental disorder known as Rett syndrome that left her with a profound intellectual disability, a number of physical handicaps, and epilepsy. She could not speak, had extremely limited mobility, and spent her days in a tilt/recline wheelchair with a headrest and seatbelt. "Jane," sixty-four and an institution resident for fifty-two years, had bipolar disorder as well as a profound intellectual disability. She had cataracts in both eyes, arthritis, and a history of hurting herself and others — headbanging, hitting and headbutting others, throwing objects, smearing feces, vomiting, and bullying. And she screamed — 103 times a day, on average — when she was unhappy.

Finding suitable physical spaces for the individuals in the case studies was hard enough, but that was only part of the process. The social needs of each resident — from day programs to entertainment opportunities, to diet, to how they liked to spend their down time — also had to be taken into account. Otherwise, the province risked a repetition of the problems that plagued the homes for special care program of the 1970s.

This time, with some exceptions, the province got things more or less right.

The Brock researchers found that the vast majority of former institution residents — over 90 per cent — ended up in group homes that had been specially adapted for their particular needs. Roughly one-third of the homes had three residents or fewer, and another 59 per cent had seven or fewer residents.[50] The agencies operating the facilities reported that the quality of life of 91 per cent of the individuals was good or excellent.

Overall, most of the former residents' well-being in the community was as good as or better than it had been in the institutions. Their physical health was stable or improved, their mental health was variable but largely improved, they had better chances to make choices about how to spend their time, and many were able to take part in community activities. Family members of the residents — only a small minority actually had family members — reported similarly positive results.[51]

One hundred and twenty or so of the last remaining Rideau Regional residents, in total, wound up in Ottawa. By 2009, twenty-three new group homes had been built in the city, and fifteen others expanded, but the moves irritated some Ottawa families who already had developmentally disabled children living at home. They complained that the Rideau Regional transfers were making it more and more difficult to secure a place for their own children. The wait list for a spot in a group home in the Ottawa area had five hundred names on it that spring. The community and social services minister, Madeleine Meilleur, insisted that the Rideau Regional closing had nothing to do with the growing wait list, and the costs of closing came from a different financial envelope. But that didn't help the families who had to wait, some for years, for a placement.[52]

Finally, inevitably, closing day arrived. The Southwestern Regional Centre shut down on October 31, 2008. The largest of the three, Rideau Regional, and the oldest, Huronia, closed at the end of March 2009. There was little fanfare and even less celebration.

On the final day at Rideau Regional, about seventy former staff members gathered in the administrative office to reunite with former co-workers, share stories, and remember their clients who had become friends. A more formal gathering that night in nearby Brockville struck a more sombre tone. The crowd celebrated the idea that no one in Ontario would ever be put into an institution simply for having a developmental disability, and prayed that everyone with a disability would be loved and respected for who they were. A candlelight vigil remembered all those who died in the institutions, those who were released, and the staff members who cared for them.

A number of speakers reflected on their experiences in institutional care. Gordon Ferguson, president of the Brockville branch of the national disability advocacy group People First, described the sixteen years he spent at Rideau Regional as a nightmare. Before he was released in 1974, he made thirteen attempts to escape. He still feels traumatized. "Every time I talk about this I have nightmares," Ferguson said. "I wish that I can get this out of my mind." David McKillop, who spent twenty years at Rideau Regional and still bears the scars, said he was "very happy" to see the place close. "I've seen so many people go through the problems like I did," he said.[53]

Gone is not forgotten. Scars fade but never disappear. And McKillop would soon get a chance to share his story, and his scars, with a far wider audience.

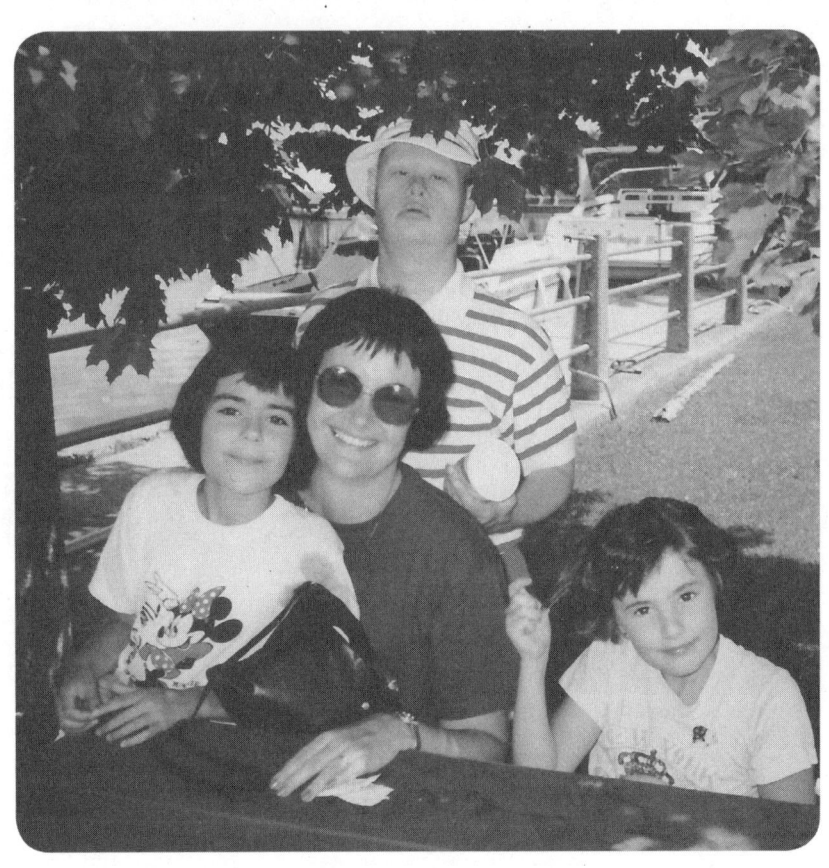

Convincing my mother to let my daughters, Rosemary (left) and Madeline (right), meet Bill took a lot of work, but it paid off for everyone.

Chapter 10

"RED FLAGGED"

Secrets run like ivy along the branches of my father's family tree, spreading wide and from one generation to the next. Large or small, members of my father's family have kept them all with stinging ferocity. It drove my mother crazy, but the roots of the habit go deep.

I learned a good one from my cousins just a few years ago: after my grandfather Bert walked out on Bessie and their sons, he apparently had not one but two other families. Dad, who cut Bert out of his life long before having his own children, knew about one of those families, but rarely talked to us about it. In fact, Dad rarely talked about his father at all, and needless to say we never met him. As we grew older, Bessie would sometimes tell us Bert secrets, usually in a whisper and always followed by an order: "Don't tell!" Bert had an affair with the family maid, right under Bessie's nose. Bert ran off with money from the bank he managed. Bert smuggled liquor to the United States during Prohibition. Who knows whether these were real events, or wisps of memories that grew more fantastical as the years passed. Other family secrets were less exotic but guarded just as fiercely. A distant relative's unnamed sorrow, referred to frequently but obliquely in the Stuart family history (it turns out her hair had fallen out). A cousin's secret wedding. A great-aunt's cancer, known only to her doctor. Details of Uncle John's final illness, confided to my father but no one else.

Dad's people were Scottish-Canadian settlers — tough, stoic, and proud, dismissive of weakness in others and anxious to hide any weaknesses of their own. Keeping secrets — or, at least, not telling the full truth — preserved the image they wanted to project. But my father's urge toward secrecy also had a gentler side. He almost never complained about the bad things in his life: not about his health (which was amazingly good until suddenly it wasn't), or the loss of his wife, or the pain of being abandoned by his father, or the horrors he saw in the war, or the terror he felt when his daughter and then his granddaughter were diagnosed with cancer. One of his closest friends described him as emotionally constipated. But as he saw it, if you can't solve a problem, why bother others with it? What good does it do to make other people worry, or feel as bad as you? Better to smile and carry on.

So I guess it shouldn't surprise me that when it came to Bill, Dad and Mom kept a whopper of a secret: Bill had infectious hepatitis B for most of his life. By the spring of 1995, when he was thirty-eight, his liver was shot.

Bill had more than his fair share of health problems over the years, including a heart murmur, a seizure that may or may not have been epilepsy, several bouts of pneumonia and bronchitis, a thyroid condition, and countless staph infections and abscesses. My sister, Mary, recalls Dad telling her Bill had had hepatitis when he was very young and living at Smiths Falls. A blood test taken much later indicating hepatitis A antibodies suggests this was probably true, but I found nothing else in his institutional record about this. Given how skimpy the records from the 1960s are in his personal file, though, the lack of information does not necessarily mean anything. I was able to find out that his hepatitis B infection occurred before he was nineteen and that, once he contracted that virus, he was never able to get rid of it.

I found the details in a four-page record of immunization and tests, running from 1960 to 1995. It reports a blood test taken in February 1975 and notes the result as "hepatitis B antigen positive." This means Bill had an active infection, though whether it was a new one or a chronic infection is impossible to tell. More blood tests were taken in 1976 and 1979, but the place on the form where the results should be recorded is blank. In March of 1980 he got a gamma globulin shot, which was commonly given at Rideau Regional during hepatitis outbreaks but was also used as an immune system booster. There's no explanation of why he got the shot: simply a record that he'd had one. Six months later, a blood test found both antigens and antibodies for hepatitis B.

Understanding the difference between antigens and antibodies in hepatitis B cases is important. Antigens are foreign substances in the body, like the hepatitis B virus itself. Antibodies are the body's response to those antigens, and typically prevent future infections. But one form of antibody, the core antibody, does not protect against future infections. The 1980 test result indicated that, despite the presence of an antibody, his hepatitis B was still active.

In 1981, he was tested again. Again, the place where the results should be recorded is blank. However, a full lab report on those tests tucked elsewhere into his file shows he had a continuing infection. In December of 1984, three years after that 1981 test, Bill was "red flagged" at the institution as a hepatitis B carrier: someone who could pass on the disease through an exchange of blood or other bodily fluids, even though he showed no symptoms of the disease. I have no idea why it took three years for him to be flagged, and shudder to think that he might have infected anyone else during those years.

Certainly, though, Bill's hepatitis was anything but an isolated case. Hepatitis, an acute liver infection caused by a virus, was widespread at all the institutions for people with intellectual disabilities, in Canada and elsewhere. Especially during the years of Bill's childhood, residents lived in overcrowded wards, ate in overcrowded cafeterias, shared showers and bathrooms, washed and brushed their teeth together, and roughhoused with each other. Some were never fully toilet trained. Many had a limited ability to keep themselves clean, and everyone had limited access to baths and showers. So it is no surprise that hepatitis A, spread when someone ingests contaminated fecal particles from a person who has the infection, ran rampant.

Between the 1950s and 1970s, the Willowbrook State School in New

York was the site of research into how the disease spread and the effective-
ness of gamma globulin in combatting it. As part of this research, doctors
deliberately infected new residents—all of them children, aged three to
ten—with live hepatitis virus. The researchers justified their work on the
grounds that almost all of these new residents would have come down
with hepatitis anyway, so infecting them was acceptable. The parents of
the children involved consented to the experiment, though there is some
question about whether they were fully informed of the risk and whether
agreeing to the experiment was a condition for getting their children into
Willowbrook. Word of these experiments triggered a public outcry, and
accusations that the researchers were using the most vulnerable children
as guinea pigs. The case is still discussed in classes on biomedical ethics.[1]

A critical outcome of the research, however, was that the researchers
concluded there were different strains of the disease, hepatitis A and
B, and that they spread in different ways. (The hepatitis C virus was
discovered later, in 1989. Since then, D and E strains have also been
identified.) Hepatitis A spreads by consuming contaminated food or
drink or by touching a contaminated surface, like a door knob or a
stairway railing, and putting your finger in your mouth later. Hepatitis
B infection happens when the blood, semen, or other bodily fluids of an
infected person enter another person's body. This can happen through
shared needles or razors, bites that break the skin, cuts sewn shut with
improperly sterilized needles, or through sex or childbirth. At one time
the disease was known as serum hepatitis, reflecting how it's transmitted.
People who contract hepatitis B often have few or no symptoms and can
pass the disease along to someone else without knowing they've done so.
It is extremely infectious.

Dad told me, near the end of his own life, that bad medical practice
at the institution caused Bill's hepatitis. He believed Bill contracted it
during a round of routine immunization shots against other diseases.
The picture he painted was of medical personnel lining up children, and
poking one child after another without changing the needle. If one had

an infection, those next in line would be exposed to it, too. I don't know where he got this idea, or even when my parents learned about Bill's hepatitis. Like so much else about Bill, Dad talked about it reluctantly and only when asked directly; even then, his answers were typically short and often vague. When I asked him how long he had known about Bill's hepatitis, Dad replied, "A while." That's all he would say.

Most people who get hepatitis B recover on their own, but about one in ten develops a chronic infection. The younger someone is when infected with hepatitis B, the more likely that individual is to develop the chronic form of the disease. According to the US Hepatitis B Foundation, more than 90 per cent of infants and up to 50 per cent of children five and under who contract hepatitis B end up with chronic infections. Most, though able to give the disease to someone else, are not ill themselves. But according to the World Health Organization, between 20 and 30 per cent of adults with chronic hepatitis B infections go on to develop cirrhosis or liver cancer.[2]

In the mid-seventies, the province decided to survey institution residents to get a sense of just how big a problem hepatitis B posed. The results were shocking. The survey found that between 70 and 80 per cent of Huronia residents either had, or had recovered from, hepatitis B. Similar levels showed up at Rideau Regional. Residents with Down syndrome had higher hepatitis B infection rates than anyone else, with a cumulative prevalence at Rideau Regional of 91 per cent. They were also more likely than other residents to be carriers of the disease: at Rideau Regional, 27 per cent of residents with Down syndrome had hepatitis B antigens compared to 6 per cent of other residents; at Huronia, 30 per cent of residents with Down syndrome were carriers.[3] Bill's hepatitis test in 1975 was probably part of this study.

The Down syndrome link is curious, and I came across a couple of possible explanations for it. Probably the most convincing was that children with Down syndrome tended to be admitted to the institutions at a younger age than other residents—in my brother's case, at two and a half—and therefore were exposed to the disease earlier, more often, and over a longer period of time than residents who were admitted in their teens or as adults. If Dad was correct, this means that Bill's chances of acquiring hepatitis B during a routine childhood immunization would also be higher, simply because he had most of his immunization shots at the institution. And if Bill had become infected before the age of five, he would have had a 50 per cent chance of becoming a carrier. A number of researchers have found that people with Down syndrome have abnormalities in their immune systems, raising the possibility that they are more likely to come down with diseases. Recent studies, however, show that people with Down syndrome who have not been institutionalized have the same incidence of hepatitis B as the rest of us—they are no more and no less likely to get it than anyone else.[4]

—

Western medicine is pretty good at preventing epidemics or limiting infection when one threatens to break out. If the medical staff at the institutions knew hepatitis was a problem—and certainly they did—then the question is why they were unable to contain it. A handful of documents in the Archives of Ontario about outbreaks in the 1960s provide some clues. In line with medical science at the time, these reports make no distinction between hepatitis A and the hepatitis B strain that Bill had. But they reveal some remarkable lapses in care, and say a great deal about the conditions of institutional life.

Between 1955 and 1961, 259 Rideau Regional residents were diagnosed with infectious hepatitis. The worst year was 1958, when 135 people contracted the disease.[5] Only seven cases were reported in 1960, but the disease rebounded in 1961, when forty-three residents and three staff became sick. A report on the 1961 outbreak details a stunning and varied series of medical errors:

- the medical staff decided to give residents immune-boosting shots of gamma globulin, but were uncertain about the right dose;

- the institution ran short of gamma globulin in the men's ward where the first case occurred, so only some of the people who lived there received injections;
- after a case cropped up in a women's ward, the medical orders to inoculate everyone else on the ward went missing for some time;
- anyone who came down with the disease was supposed to be sent to an isolation ward but, when the isolation ward filled up, some were treated on their home wards, which "considerably increased the likelihood of infection";
- a boy who was released back to his ward after time in isolation was later found to still have an active case of hepatitis;
- after a very young girl in the nursery ward fell ill, everyone else on the ward was inoculated—except for one little girl who was away at the time, and then ended up getting the disease;
- three residents developed hepatitis after getting their gamma globulin shots; and
- five residents who got routine booster shots on the same day later came down with hepatitis, though seventy others who got the shots that day did not.

The report concluded, however, that the main source of the spread was direct, person-to-person contact.[6]

A draft report dated February 26, 1962—apparently a second post-mortem on the 1961 outbreak—found more problems. One patient had developed symptoms after a transfer from the special treatment unit, and the ward staff concluded he picked it up there. The nurse in charge of the special treatment unit, however, "emphatically denied" that anyone in the unit had the disease. Some residents may have missed their gamma globulin shots, or received incorrect dosages, because the paperwork on who was to receive what dose was kept in the office. The staff recalculated doses once they got to a ward and, as a result, "there was no check that all patients received the gamma globulin and no check that they received the dose recorded in the office." This 1962 report says that staff followed proper procedures in administering the shots. Initially, they gave shots to the buttock. Given that many residents weren't toilet trained, this raised an unsettling possibility: "If the buttock were contaminated by feces, it would theoretically be possible to introduce the virus with the injection." The medical staff decided to give injections to the arm in future. Arm or buttock, the syringe was detached after each shot and placed in an antiseptic solution, then washed and sterilized in a machine known as an autoclave. The report said, however, that the autoclave should be checked to see whether it was working properly. Meanwhile, in the kitchen, the dietician was reported to be "quite upset about the prevalence of hepatitis in her staff, especially her cooks."[7] The idea of food handlers with active cases of hepatitis is stomach-churning.

A health inspection in April 1962 found a range of hygiene problems that could also have contributed to the spread of the disease. In some wards, dishes were washed on the same slabs used to hose down patients. In some resident dining rooms, urine or feces had to be wiped up from the chairs and floor after every meal. "I was told that staff members cleaned it up but since there is such a staff shortage it is inconceivable that patients don't have some contact with the contaminated material," the inspector wrote. "The same patients then proceed to dry and distribute the dishes and cutlery." To keep plastic glasses from breaking, the water temperature in the dishwashers was set below the recommended level, which meant dishes and cutlery were not properly cleaned. Some residents working in the dining halls had poor hygiene: "One patient was observed to pick his nose, scratch himself, and then distribute the milk pitchers by insertion of his hand into the pitcher rather than holding it by the handle." The inspector noted that the medical staff were conducting a mass TB survey by using a "flame-sterilized needle" rather than separate syringes. The inspector concluded that while person-to-person transmission was the cause in most instances, "the possibility that the virus has been introduced by a common source (contaminated needle or instrument) cannot be ruled out."[8]

Guidelines circulated in 1978 on dealing with residents with chronic hepatitis B raised other possible vectors of infection.[9] "Great care must be taken that the toothbrushes of residents be kept only for the use of the resident concerned," the guidelines say. This made me think of the bathroom scenes in the film *Danny and Nicky*: sure, each boy had his own toothbrush, but they brushed their teeth in groups at each sink, and it was messy business. The guidelines said anyone who tested positive for hepatitis B antigens should be barred from using the institution's swimming pool and be prevented from working as food handlers. Only those "whose hygiene habits are well established," it said, should be allowed to look after smaller children. The institution also came up with rules to ensure doctors or dentists were fully informed if a resident needing treatment had hepatitis B.

In short, though I found nothing in the provincial archive or Bill's file to substantiate Dad's description of how Bill became infected, I found nothing to disprove it either. Instead, I discovered any number of ways Bill could have been infected, and even more ways he could have been protected against infection. I also found any number of ways he might have passed the disease on to other people.

Dad told me he was so angry when he and Mom learned about Bill's hepatitis status that they considered taking legal action against the Rideau Regional Centre. In the end, they decided not to. A lawsuit wouldn't make any difference to Bill, he said, and it wouldn't make him better. What good, he and Mom asked themselves, would it do to make a fuss about it? None, they decided.

This was all news to me. Mary, Bob, and I had no idea Bill had hepatitis B until the very last week of his life.

—

By the mid-seventies, Mary, Bob, and I had all left home. Mary studied archeology in Toronto, met her future husband on a dig in Egypt, and moved to New York in 1979. Bob studied geography at York University in Toronto and worked in a number of places before finding his calling, in 1990, as a professor in Australia and Hong Kong. I worked for an Ottawa newspaper for a year after graduating. My work took me to Toronto, Washington, Philadelphia, and Kingston, Ontario. I didn't see Bill for several years, and knew from talking with Mom that he was fragile. When I saw him again after moving back to Ottawa in 1987, I was surprised at how old he looked — far older than someone in his early thirties should. His hair had been patchy for years, but now he was almost completely bald. His face was wizened and criss-crossed with lines, wrinkles, and old scars. His teeth were worn down from years of grinding. He complained loudly about climbing up or down stairs, whether from pain or fear of falling I could not tell. He moved stiffly, like an old man. Nonetheless, he was still Bill, still the same sweet and goofy guy he had always been. I don't know whether he recognized me — probably not, after years apart — but he was glad to see me. At one point during our first visit, he swatted me on the head, said, "Nice haircut!" and cackled with laughter. This was an old and favourite joke, and it made me laugh, too.

I saw him several times in the 1980s and early 1990s. I would have visited more often, but Mom took on the role of gatekeeper and discouraged it. In a way, I understood her reluctance. I knew that she and Bill enjoyed the private routines of their monthly visits, and that Bill found changes in his routine upsetting. And, as he entered his middle thirties, she and Dad were becoming more and more worried that something else would erase what little they had left of him.

They were worried about Alzheimer's disease.

The link between Down syndrome and Alzheimer's was well established by the 1990s, though the science behind the link was — and is — still being investigated. By the time they are forty, studies have found, virtually everyone with Down syndrome shows some of the brain changes characteristic of Alzheimer's. At the age of thirty-five, one in four has Alzheimer's-type dementia; by the age of sixty-five, it's three out of four.[10] The staff at Rideau Regional had been aware of this problem and had, in fact, enrolled Bill in a study of dementia, obsessive-compulsive behaviour, and Down syndrome.[11]

In early 1994, after many years without any sign of epilepsy, Bill had a seizure. His doctors admitted him to the infirmary and started him on a common anti-seizure medication, carbamazepine. Over the next six months, his mental condition deteriorated sharply. In his monthly report for September, one of his counsellors wrote: "Not a great month. Bill extremely non-compliant. Appears ill at certain times but at others can be accused of attempting to con the staff." Other reports that fall noted he was shaky, lethargic, and tired. After seeing Bill in October, his doctor wrote: "Presently, according to his counsellor, he is quite independent in terms of self help and domestic skills. On the other hand he doesn't seem to concentrate well and needs to be told 'over and over' to do things. There is a question as to whether this might be 'attention seeking' — this is a possibility given his general behavioral pattern over the years. On the other hand he is perseverative and very slow in doing things, suggestive of dementia. . . . The development of seizures is suggestive of the onset of dementia but we will just have to observe in terms of follow up if there is significant deterioration."

Mom noticed during her monthly visits that year that Bill seemed disoriented, disengaged, or, as she put it to me one day after a visit, "dopey." The staff reported that his balance was off. His fine-motor skills had deteriorated to the point where he had trouble holding a fork or a crayon. Given that eating and colouring were two of his favourite activities, this must have been deeply frustrating for him. He had crying spells for no apparent reason, sometimes during the day and sometimes in the middle of the night. He fell asleep at meals. He got lost on the grounds of the institution, something he had never done before. He didn't recognize people he should have recognized. He seemed depressed. He lost interest in social outings. Bill had always been slow to do things like shaving or getting dressed, but now it took him ages to complete even the simplest task.

His doctor suspected Bill's problem was Alzheimer's. The psychologist at the Alzheimer's clinic disagreed. "Dementia may be developing but it is curious that he appears to have progressed from no dementia to the last stages in less than a year's time," he wrote in December of that year. Dad, putting his medical training and his contacts with medical experts to good use, wondered whether the problem might be the epilepsy medication itself—perhaps Bill was over-medicated or having a toxic reaction to carbamazepine. Dad talked with Bill's doctor in December, and asked him to take Bill off carbamazepine and switch to another medication. The doctor agreed. As soon as he started to decrease the dose, however, Bill had a seizure.

Bill spent several weeks in the infirmary at the end of that year, during which he was weaned off carbamazepine and moved over to another anti-seizure drug, valproic acid. When he was discharged, his medical file listed the "final diagnosis" as Alzheimer's disease, a possible sensitivity to carbamazepine, and seizures. Strangely, given that he had been red flagged since 1981 as a hepatitis B carrier, there was no mention of the possibility that a failing liver might have played a role in his illness. In fact, I am not sure his doctor even knew of his hepatitis B status. A note written in his medical file in early 1995 referred to a 1991 test showing he was "antibody positive"—cured, in other words. I found that 1991 result on his record of immunization and tests, with a brief note saying "status change." The conclusion that he no longer had an active hepatitis B infection was, however, incorrect. Tests in 1992 and beyond confirmed an active infection. His doctor, it appears, did not pick up on the later results.

The change in medication seemed to work. The seizures stopped, and Bill was more mentally alert, but some troubling physical problems persisted. One was swelling, especially of his face, legs, ankles, and feet. Another was a low white blood cell count. He was also deeply fatigued. All three are signs of liver damage, but no one made that connection.

He was seen at the psychiatric clinic in February 1995, following up on his behaviour over the last year. The notes on that appointment report a heartbreaking incident: "In the clinic he is quite animated and from time to time points to his abdomen and legs as if they are providing some kind of discomfort. At one point, he lay down on the floor in what appears to be an attention-seeking effort." Clearly, Bill was trying to tell the doctor something, but the message did not get through. The staff member who accompanied him thought he was acting out to get attention. "Billy was in a good frame of mind. He acted like a HAM, lying on the floor face down. Doctor M___ found Billy to be quite the LAD."[12] The doctor's conclusion was that Bill didn't seem to have either dementia or depression.

What Bill had, it turns out, was end-stage cirrhosis, but it would be months before anybody figured that out. He fell ill again at the end of March 1995, with what the admission notes say were a fever and cough, and was sent back to the infirmary. His seizures were under control, but he didn't seem to be tolerating the new anti-seizure medication terribly well so the doctor switched him to another medication, Dilantin, with Lasix to reduce the swelling. Two liver function tests done as part of his blood work found levels out of the normal range, and his random glucose level was also off. All are possible signs of cirrhosis, but his doctor only underlined the glucose result and wrote a one-word note beside it: "Why?" The nursing notes say he had a lot of swelling in his legs and feet, which got worse over the next month. His belly was swollen, and so was his face. He was slow, shaky, and pale.

In April his doctor referred him to a specialist. The referral note, like so many other things in his file, has an error; it lists Bill's age as forty-eight, not thirty-eight. But the doctor had finally made the hepatitis connection. His referral (the spelling errors and underlining are in the original) read: "This man is a chronic hepatitis B <u>carrier</u>. I suspect his is incipient liver <u>failure</u> due to chirrosis. He is red flagged a Hep B carrier but was antibody positive in 1991. <u>Will recheck status and d/c red flag if wrong</u>. Fairly recent check says antigen positive."

On April 27, Bill's doctor noted the bad news from the specialist (again, the errors are in the original medical record): "Dr. C____ feel liver almost totally destroyed with cirrhosis. No really much to be done."

—

On the afternoon of April 27, 1995, I came home from work and noticed the message light on our answering machine was blinking. A doctor from Rideau Regional had left a long and convoluted message, but the gist was clear and shocking, at least to me: Bill was in the infirmary. His liver was failing. His condition was terminal, and he was being put on palliative care. The doctor was calling me because Mom and Dad were away — they were in California but due back soon — and I was their emergency contact.

I immediately phoned the doctor to get more details and to discuss what we should do. Bill was dying, he said, but he was well medicated and not in a lot of pain. I told him I understood that he couldn't predict how long Bill would live, but Mom and Dad would be devastated if Bill died while they were away. How perilous, I asked, was his condition? The doctor told me that his best guess was that Bill would live for a couple more weeks. I asked for his advice on what to do about my parents. Should I call them? Should I tell them to come home? He had no answers. I could call them if I wished, he said, or I could let them enjoy their vacation. Bill will probably still be here when they get back, he added.

I was still processing the news when my husband, Vinny, came home. I played him the phone message and, as I listened to it a second time, I felt a flash of anger. The essence of the message was *Hi, sorry you're not home, your brother's dying, call me.* Really? Who leaves a message like that on a family answering machine? Why not simply leave a message asking me to call the doctor at Rideau Regional? The answering machine sat in the dining room and took calls for all of us. My kids, then fourteen and twelve, routinely checked it. How would they have reacted if they'd heard that message?

I swallowed my anger. If the doctor was insensitive or arrogant, there was nothing I could do about that. But there were other things I could do.

First, I phoned Mom and Dad to let them know what was going on. This was a tougher decision than it sounds. Mom was about to turn seventy-five and had a weak heart. They really wanted, and probably needed, this trip after a long, cold Ottawa winter. But the news about Bill wasn't something I could keep secret. If Bill died while they were away, and I hadn't told them I knew he was terminal, I would never forgive myself. I caught them the afternoon before they were to head to the Grand Canyon. They said they would cut their trip short and come home.

Second, I decided to go and see for myself how Bill was doing. Vinny and I headed to Smiths Falls the next morning, stopping at the Burger King on the way to pick up a milkshake. I figured Bill might like it and find it easier to digest than his usual hamburger. We drove over to Rideau Regional, along the roads I had travelled so many times, checked in at the desk, and walked the long corridors to the infirmary. Unlike when we were children, the corridors were pretty much deserted. By this time, most of the residents had been moved out. Those left were people like Bill—adults, not children; lifers who, for any number of reasons, hadn't been moved to a spot in the community.

We found Bill propped up in a bed, alert and in pretty good spirits, and happy to have company. He sipped the milkshake, though he could swallow only a bit of it. I told him Mom and Dad would be coming to see him as soon as they got home from their trip. He smiled and nodded. Vinny told Bill he heard that Bill really liked hamburgers. Was that true? Bill perked up instantly. "Hamburger," he said and nodded. Vinny asked, did he like french fries, too? Again, Bill nodded. "French fries," he said then looked around to see if we had brought any with us. I asked the nurse if it would be okay if we went and got him a hamburger and fries. We didn't want to make him sicker, but if a burger wouldn't do any damage, we'd like to get him one. She said she didn't think that was a good idea. So we stayed.

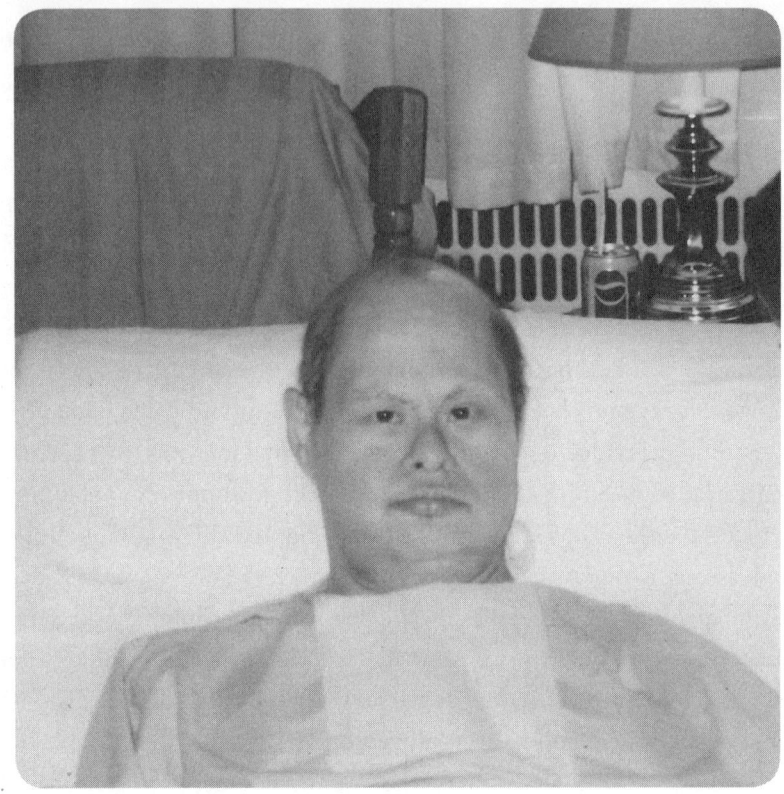

My parents were away when Bill's liver condition became terminal,
but they made it home in time to be with him for his final days.
Dad took this picture of Bill just days before his death.

I wish now that we had got him that burger. It would have been a
small kindness for a man whose life lacked so many small kindnesses.

We stayed for an hour or so, talking to Bill and the nurses caring for
him. The conversation with Bill was mostly one-way, as always; it's hard
to talk with someone whose spoken vocabulary is limited to a dozen
words. The people caring for him seemed attentive, and Bill didn't seem
to be in pain. The doctor dropped by and filled us in on Bill's condition
and the palliative care plan. Without asking Bill's permission, he flipped
back the covers so we could see Bill's legs. They were horribly swollen. So
was his belly. After a while, it was clear Bill was getting tired. I reminded

him that Mom would come to see him soon, and again he smiled and nodded. I kissed him goodbye, and Vinny and I headed home.

We picked Mom and Dad up at the airport the next night. After a few hours of sleep they headed to the Rideau Regional Centre. Mom phoned to say Bill looked pretty good and was very happy to see them. Mom cuddled him and patted him, fluffed his pillows and rubbed lotion on his hands and feet, and gave him sips of apple juice with an ice cube in it — all the things she did for us when we were kids and were down with a cold or the flu. No one was better at taking care of a sick child than Mom, and Bill must have loved it. He's smiling in the photograph Dad took of him and Mom that day, the last one anyone would ever take of him. Mom and Dad came home that night and went back the next morning, settling into a room for families of residents who were terminally ill. I drove out to join them for a couple of hours. I didn't ask Mom if I could come; she probably would have said no if I had. I simply went.

Bill looked much worse. He had severe swelling of his stomach, legs, face, and feet. The skin on his back and buttocks was blistered. His temperature was up. He was on morphine for pain and barely conscious. It was clear he was dying. The medical file for May 3 notes, somewhat ominously, that he had "survived the night." He wouldn't survive the next one. He lost consciousness around noon. His colour was bad. His blood pressure sagged. His pulse fell. He stopped breathing for brief periods. Eventually, he stopped breathing altogether. He was pronounced dead around four a.m. on May 4, 1995.

—

If giving birth to a child with Down syndrome in the 1950s presented social complications, burying that child in the 1990s had its own complexities.

Our parents, who grew up at a time when the dead were laid out in open caskets in the family parlour, were grateful for the modern funeral home. And, like most families, we had routines that carried us through those first days of bereavement. Typically, we made the funeral arrangements, put a notice on the obituary page of the local paper, and scheduled visitation hours for the afternoon and evening before the funeral. These were times when people could gather and talk and sympathize, but no one could overstay their welcome or raid the liquor cabinet. Mom had a horror of open caskets, so the casket was always closed. A Protestant minister officiated at family funerals, and we kept the services short and personal, with a few favourite hymns, a Bible reading or two (usually Psalm 23), and a eulogy from someone from the family. A reception followed the service—coffee, tea, finger sandwiches, hors d'oeuvres, cookies—either at the funeral home or at the house of one family member or another.

With Billy, things were different, as they always were.

It didn't make sense to have the funeral in Ottawa. Bill knew almost no one in Ottawa aside from his immediate family, and almost no one in Ottawa knew Bill. It made no more sense to hold the funeral in the town of Smiths Falls. He knew little of Smiths Falls aside from the Burger King, the shops on Beckwith Street, the park, the drugstore, the grocery store, and the chocolate factory. His world was the tightly closed community of the Rideau Regional Centre.

The staff at the centre lined up a local funeral home to handle the arrangements and a pleasant, round-faced, young Baptist minister to conduct the service in an assembly room at Rideau Regional. He had never met Bill, and Mary recalls that he wasn't the regular chaplain for the institution. But he was available, accommodating, and caring, and very kindly came to meet Mom and Dad at the institution the day before Bill died. Mom told him she wanted a closed casket but otherwise left things to him.

On the day of the funeral, the family gathered in a private room at Rideau Regional before the service. We were a small group: Mom and Dad; Mary and her husband, Richard, up from New York; Vinny and me, along with our daughters, Rosemary and Madeline. Bob was living in Australia and couldn't make it home. The minister joined us and suggested leading us in a family prayer for Bill's soul, confident we would agree. Dad smiled, gave a small shrug, and nodded. Mom stiffened. "No," she said. She did not want to say that kind of prayer. The minister, taken aback, stammered a bit. He then suggested that we are all God's children and that after we die our souls fly up to join God in Heaven. This is a wonderful thing and Bill's soul was worth praying for; surely Mom believed this was so, he prompted her gently.

Again, Mom's response surprised me: "No." She said she didn't believe in life after death. When you die, she said, you die. Religion had always been one of those agree-to-disagree issues between Mom and Dad and, of the two, Mom had been the more devout. We went to church every Sunday when we were children, but that was Mom's doing, not Dad's. Dad liked the ceremony and the socializing of Sunday services and was happy to go along when he didn't have a golf game or a curling game or a day of skiing lined up, or when he wasn't on call, but he was not particularly interested in the deeper questions of faith and divinity. Mom, on the other hand, periodically threw herself into religious study, taking courses and reading books as she tried to come to terms with aspects of the faith she found hard to accept. After the rest of us stopped going to church except on holidays, Mom became a Sunday school teacher. But somewhere along the way, I guess, she had lost her faith, and none of us had known.

Family prayer left unsaid, the minister ushered us into an assembly room. Aunt Lois, Mom and Dad's sister-in-law who used to visit Bill occasionally with Mom, was there. Her son, David, and his wife, Rosalind, had driven her and were sitting with her, but that was it for people from outside the institution. Everyone else was part of Bill's community: residents, counsellors, staff members. The provincial Report of Institutional Burial form, filled out by the company that handled the funeral, noted "78 friends + relatives" attended. That number surprises Mary and me. Neither of us remembers more than a few dozen people there, though to be fair we weren't counting.

As we moved toward our seats, one of Bill's former counsellors, a young woman I had met a few times and liked, pulled me aside. She said she knew the family wanted a closed casket, but asked if we would agree to open it at the end of the service so Bill's friends could say goodbye. Otherwise they might not understand he was really gone. I told her that sounded like a good and thoughtful idea and said I would talk to Mom. Mom, after hardly a moment's pause, agreed.

The service was short and simple. A few Bible readings. A prayer or two. No hymns. A brief homily from the minister, who promised that Heaven was real, as real as any house on any street, and so real that it might as well have an address. (I could feel Mom and Mary gritting their teeth at that one.) There was no family eulogy. No tears from the family either; a few from his friends and the staff.

When the casket was opened after the service, his friends walked up, one by one, and peered inside. These were probably some of the same people I tried not to stare at as children, when Mom and Dad moved Bill into the hospital school. They were older and greyer, the years worn hard on their faces and bodies. Most of them didn't say anything; they simply looked at Bill, nodded, and headed out of the room. Others spoke their goodbyes. When one said, "So long, Boo," my heart jumped — I had completely forgotten until that moment that Boo was the nickname we had given him all those years ago, before he left us. A few people said, "Bye, Bill." A woman my daughter Madeline spotted earlier — Madeline was shocked to see that the woman was wearing no panties under her dress — leaned over and kissed him on the cheek. A man hooted and gave an exuberant wave as he left the room, calling out loudly, "Bye-bye."

It was a small send-off, but Bill was destined from his birth to live a small life. Our family made sure of that, and so did the institution where he lived. Bill didn't have a chance to have much impact on the world. But he did, eventually, have a home of sorts at Rideau Regional, and the people who shared it with him would miss him.

Mom and Dad put a death notice in the local paper the day after the funeral. It was brief, saying Bill had died peacefully at the institution at the age of thirty-eight, and the funeral service had already been held. It ended this way: "The family wish to express our heartfelt thanks to the staff at Rideau Regional Centre for their loving care and devotion to our Bill. Please—no floral or memorial gifts."

We buried him in the double plot Mom and Dad had bought for themselves at Pinecrest Cemetery in Ottawa. As we drove away from the cemetery, Mom looked out the car window, gave a little wave, and whispered, "Goodbye, Bill." Mary, who was in the car with her and Dad, says that moment was the saddest and most touching moment of the day.

A few weeks after Bill's death, the institution sent Mom and Dad a letter. Its sole content was a consent-to-treatment form for Bill. Mom scrawled a large double X across the form and wrote, "Our son died at Rideau Regional on May 4/95 and was buried from your chapel on May 5/95." She signed it and printed her name as "Mrs. Douglas McKercher," adding "Dr. +" before "Mrs." as an afterthought, and sent it back. On June 14, the administrator sent her a note apologizing for the mistake. "We know that in sending out over 900 forms we are bound to commit errors. However we feel particularly upset about this one." I am sure she did. But how hard it would have been to get it right in the first place?

—

Mom died the following winter, and we buried her in the plot beside Bill. It seemed right, somehow, that the child she had given up in life should lie next to her in death. When Dad died fifteen years later, we cremated his body and buried the ashes between the two of them, in a bamboo box designed to disintegrate. I like to think that whatever remains of the three of them has mingled together in that small piece of land, settling into the earth as one.

Chapter 11

"AN AIR OF **VIOLENCE** AND **PUNISHMENT**"

The final chapter in the story of the large Ontario residential institutions began more than a decade after Bill and Mom died. By the time it came to a close in late 2013, Dad was gone, too. That was, in a way, a kindness. Had Dad been alive, he would have had to admit that the decades-old article of faith in my family, that sending Bill to Smiths Falls was the best thing we could have done for him, was deeply, fundamentally, cruelly wrong. Acknowledging this was hard enough for Bob, Mary, and me. For our parents, it would have been devastating.

This part of the story begins, as most things relating to these institutions do, at the Huronia Regional Centre in Orillia. That's where Marilyn Dolmage's younger brother Robert Sidey—like Bill, he had Down syndrome—died at the age of eight from untreated pneumonia. Dolmage became a social worker and worked at Huronia in the late 1960s and early 1970s, gaining a deeper understanding of the place where her brother, and thousands of others like him, spent their days. "They had all of their citizenship rights stripped away," she later told the *Globe and Mail*. "They had no control over their lives."[1] She watched staff tranquilize residents, keep them in caged cots, and spray them with a hose after meals. After leaving Huronia, Dolmage kept in touch with some former residents, including Marie Slark and Pat Seth.

As *Toronto Star* columnist Carol Goar tells it, Slark and Seth talked about their constrained, difficult, and violence-filled lives at Huronia one evening over dinner at the Dolmages' home.[2] It struck Marilyn's husband,

Jim, that their experience was not all that different from the experiences of Aboriginal children in Canada's residential school system. The residential schools, funded by the federal government and administered by various Christian denominations, took generations of children away from their families, sometimes by force, in the name of assimilating them into mainstream Canadian society. The schools deprived Aboriginal children of language and culture, family and community; many children were physically or sexually abused; and at least six thousand died while within their walls, mostly from disease. The Canadian government now recognizes the residential school program as one of the most shameful passages in Canadian history, publicly apologizing to the former residents and their communities and creating a compensation package for the roughly eighty thousand survivors.

Jim Dolmage made a videotape of Seth and Slark describing what had happened to them at Huronia in explicit detail, and he and Marilyn started looking for a lawyer to handle a class-action lawsuit. They settled on Kirk M. Baert of Koskie Minsky LLP in Toronto, one of Canada's top class-action law firms. In April 2009, just weeks after Huronia shut down, the class-action lawsuit was launched, with Seth and Slark as representatives of the class. In Ontario, people with a disability cannot act for themselves in a lawsuit, so the Dolmages became their "litigation guardians," charged with defending the interests of the plaintiffs as if those interests were their own. The class was certified the following summer, covering anyone who lived at Huronia between January 1, 1945, and March 31, 2009, and was still alive as of April 21, 2007, and their family members.[3]

Vici Clarke of Kingston, Ontario, whose family has been active in the community living movement for more than fifty years, heard about the Huronia class-action suit through an email inviting people to attend the certification hearing at Osgoode Hall, and told her mother, Muriel, and her brother, Rob, about it. Rob, who was labelled as having a developmental disability, spent ten months at Rideau Regional as a child, and he said the boys he met there also needed help. Clarke met with the

Koskie Minsky people and agreed to be involved in a Rideau Regional class-action suit as the litigation guardian for the representative plaintiff, David McKillop. McKillop, who spoke at the ceremony in Brockville to mark Rideau Regional's closing, spent twenty years at the institution. The Rideau Regional class-action suit, and one covering the Southwestern Regional Centre, were both certified in August 2011.[4]

The suits all made the same allegation: the province had failed in its duties to care for and protect the interests of people with disabilities who lived in the institutions. The suits argued that the province had been negligent in, the way it set up, funded, operated, staffed, managed, and supervised the institutions. Worse still, the government knew about the problems and failed to correct the situation. The statements of claim point out that a series of reports commissioned by and for the government, starting with Walter Williston's report in the early 1970s, detailed a range of deficiencies and injustices in the individual institutions and within the system as a whole. And yet, the statements say, the province had ignored its own advisers and failed to do what it needed to do to provide the care the residents needed.

The representative plaintiffs in the suits alleged the kinds of abuse that, in the outside world, might lead to criminal charges. Marie Slark was taken away from her family by the Children's Aid Society at the age of seven, put in foster care, and then sent to Huronia. In 1970, when she was sixteen, the institution sent her to an "approved home" off the institution grounds, where she was sexually abused. She did not report the abuse for fear of being sent back to Huronia.[5] Patricia Seth, who arrived at Huronia after being taken from her family at the age of six, endured repeated physical abuse and punishment at the institution. She said staff members hit her with a fly swatter and a brush, held her upside down in ice-cold water as punishment for not eating, and dosed her with anti-psychotic drugs as punishment for speaking out. At sixteen, Seth moved to a group home on the Huronia facility grounds, where the abuse continued. Like Slark, she was afraid to speak out for fear of retaliation.[6] David McKillop's parents dropped him off at Rideau Regional when he was almost five. He said that, when he was about eight, a staff member kicked him in the groin so hard it left him sterile. McKillop never told anyone or reported the abuse for fear of further physical retribution.[7] The representative claimant in the third class-action lawsuit, Mary Ellen Fox, was admitted to the Southwestern Regional Centre in 1971, and suffered a range of abuse. She alleged that staff robbed her of gifts from her family, locked her in a windowless room as punishment, shocked her with a cattle prod, and used medication to keep her as sedated as possible. When her family took her out of the institution in 1988, she was so drugged she couldn't walk down the stairs.[8]

McKillop's time at Rideau Regional overlapped with my brother's — he arrived four years before Bill and stayed until 1972, when Bill was sixteen — and the living conditions he describes in the statement of claim are all too familiar to anyone who had a family member living there. McKillop slept in a large dorm that was locked day and night. He had no personal possessions. He was given shoes that didn't fit.[9] The washroom stalls had no doors. He was able to shower only twice a week, and always with the other children. He had no privacy, no control over his daily life, no chance to make choices or to have any say in his daily routine. He also received virtually no education at Rideau; every year, the statement of claim said, the students were taught the same things over again. He eventually learned to read and write, but only after he'd left Rideau Regional as an adult. Instead of getting an education, he was put to work washing dishes, cleaning floors, and helping ward staff care for younger children. He was not paid for this work.

Day-to-day life was terrifying. According to the claim, Rideau Regional had "an air of violence and punishment which created significant fear among the residents and caused significant trauma." The staff fostered this atmosphere as a way of controlling the residents.[10] McKillop said he and other residents were punished, often for no reason, in humiliating and painful ways. He was ordered to clean floors or toilets with a toothbrush. He had to spend entire days dressed in a nightgown, the same punishment described by the unnamed Cedar Springs resident in the newspaper article I quoted in chapter 4. He was made to stand against a wall with his arms extended for up to two hours, or kneel and hold a pail of water in each hand. Staff and other residents, he said, physically and mentally abused him.

The most chilling part of his experience there—and the line in the statement of claim that has cost me more sleep than I'd care to admit—is this: "David repeatedly witnessed other children residing at Rideau being similarly physically punished for no reason and experienced staff members instructing minor residents to physically abuse one another at the staff's direction."[11] The idea that some staff members made children hit each other, either as punishment or for their own entertainment, suggests the wards were training grounds for bullies and enforcers, places where specific and targeted acts of violence were not only tolerated but encouraged, and even directed.

My family assumed that the new scratches and bruises we saw on Bill every time we visited him were the result of Bill's own clumsiness, or of carelessly rough but generally harmless play among the boys. After all, kids get hurt. They have accidents; they break bones now and then. But the statement of claim suggests that may have been only part of the story. Were some of Bill's scratches and bruises caused by other children acting on commands from the staff? Could Bill himself have been one of the enforcers? Bill was a tease. He liked to provoke other residents and get them in trouble. He made few friends among the residents, and he sought affection and attention from the staff. Perhaps the price Bill paid for gaining favour with the staff was bullying another child.

But even if he did not take part, simply growing up in an atmosphere that tolerated—even encouraged—this kind of violent behaviour among the residents would take a toll. In the overcrowded and understaffed wards of Bill's childhood, escape was impossible. Bill, like many other residents, didn't have the verbal skills to explain a problem like bullying or to complain in detail about abuse. His only choice was to act up.

Residents of Rideau Regional and the other institutions were either wards of the Crown or people whose care had been handed over to the

Crown. This meant, the statements of claim say, that the province owed them safe, secure, and good-quality care. And, according to the claims, the province failed on almost every level.

The Crown failed to provide adequate medical care or to report injuries. It failed to report allegations of sexual abuse, "and moreover, often punished those residents who came forward with such claims."[12] It created and fostered an atmosphere of fear and intimidation. It failed to screen job candidates adequately, or to hire staff with the appropriate qualifications, or to properly supervise activities. It failed to spend what it needed to spend on the facilities or on care of residents. It failed to respond adequately to complaints about care or to recommendations on how to improve it. It failed to safeguard the physical and emotional needs of residents.

All three statements of claim conclude with a catalogue of damages suffered by the residents during and after their stay. This one, from the Smiths Falls claim, is very similar to the Huronia one and identical to the one covering Southwestern Ontario. The list of damages reads:

(a)   emotional, physical, sexual and psychological abuse;

(b)   exacerbation of mental disability and deprivation of healing opportunities;

(c)   impairment of mental and emotional health and well-being;

(d)   an impaired ability to trust other persons;

(e)   a further impaired ability to participate in normal family affairs and relationships;

(f)   alienation from family members;

(g)   depression, anxiety, emotional stress and mental anguish;

(h)   pain and suffering;

(i)   a loss of self-esteem and feelings of humiliation and degradation;

(j)   the fact that the Rideau structure and environment was itself further disabling to those individuals, physically, emotionally and psychologically by limiting their skills and developing a learned helplessness;

(k)   a lack of and inability to gain educational and employment skills;

(l)   an impaired ability to obtain and sustain employment, resulting either in lost or reduced income and ongoing loss of income;

(m)   an impaired ability to deal with people in positions of authority;

(n)   an impaired ability to trust other individuals or sustain relationships;

(o)   a sense of isolation or separateness from their community;

(p)   a requirement for medical or psychological treatment and counselling;

(q)   an impaired ability to enjoy and participate in recreational, social and employment activities;

(r)   loss of friendship and companionship;

(s)   loss of community, social connections and the ability to develop them;

(t)   loss of opportunity to realize and exercise their citizenship rights;

(u)   sexual disorientation; and

(v)   the loss of general enjoyment of life.[13]

The suits sought billions of dollars in compensation.

The province fought back against these claims, and it fought hard. Its statement of defence against the initial lawsuit, the one covering Huronia, admitted that the Crown owned and operated the institution, and that Seth and Slark lived there. It said the Crown had no knowledge of some

of the specific points in the claim, and it denied all the others. All of
them.

Huronia, the government lawyers contended, was managed in ac-
cordance with the appropriate standards of care, even as those standards
evolved and changed. "The Crown, her employees, agents and servant,
acted at all times in the best interests of the residents of HRC," it said.[14]
Residents were not abused or traumatized. The day-to-day program at
Huronia was structured and controlled and included a variety of activities and residents participated to the extent of their abilities. Staff
were carefully selected and had the appropriate qualifications. They were
supervised on the job. "If, at any time, an allegation of mistreatment or
abuse of an HRC resident by an HRC staff member was substantiated,
the Crown took any and all appropriate steps including dismissing the
involved staff member and reporting the alleged mistreatment or abuse
to appropriate authorities."[15]

The defence statement denied allegations that the province allowed
inappropriate or unhealthy punishments, or that residents lived in an
atmosphere that threatened punishment or violence. To the extent there
were any inadequacies in the way the institution operated, "which is
expressly denied," the problems stemmed from funding decisions. These
were made "at the highest levels of government," based on competing
demands for public resources and "the government's responsibility to
taxpayers to work within approved budgets."[16]

In addition to rejecting the general allegations in the lawsuit, the
statement of defence went after some of the specific claims made by Seth
and Slark. It denied, for instance, that the "Crown has or should have
any knowledge or information about Slark's alleged mistreatment at the
approved home." It rejected Slark's claim that staff punished residents
for no reason, or instructed residents to punish each other. As for Seth,
it specifically rejected her claims of being beaten, isolated, punished for
speaking out, and drugged.[17]

It then went after the Dolmages, charging that Marilyn Dolmage
had a conflict of interest in serving as litigation guardian because she

had worked at Huronia, and that Jim Dolmage had a conflict because he was married to Marilyn. It concluded by saying nothing in the Crown's conduct warranted the award of damages to former residents, and asked that the suit be dismissed, with costs.

—

It took almost three years before a trial date was set in the Huronia case. This meant that, for three years, the class representatives and other potential witnesses had to contemplate the nerve-wracking prospect of testifying in court and being cross-examined by government lawyers. They were eager to tell their stories in public, but the wait to do so was agonizingly long. Other former residents and their families knew the case would dredge up painful memories of their own, but they did not know how or when. And, during those three years, at least six hundred former Huronia residents died. But finally a trial date was set: Monday, September 16, 2013.

On the morning of September 16, a number of former residents gathered at the courthouse in Toronto for the opening of the trial. They learned when they got there, however, that the hearing had been adjourned for twenty-four hours, with no warning and no explanation. Many former residents cried when they heard the news, fearing that their stories might never be heard. In the absence of a hearing, they talked with each other and to the media, sharing their disturbing memories. Edgar Riel, who broke down as he reacted to the delay, said that his mother had dropped him off at Huronia in the early 1960s, when he was nine. "I spent six years of hell in that place, being beat up...told that my mother had left me for good, that I was useless, a nobody," he said. "Why didn't they listen to us fifty years ago? We told them, and they just ignored us. It was our word against theirs."[18]

The reason for the delay became clear the next day: the province and the lawyers for the class had reached a settlement. Marilyn and Jim Dolmage say they had some input in shaping the final agreement—they had received a draft of the settlement the previous Friday, thought it was inadequate, and pushed for a better deal over the weekend, all afternoon and evening Monday, and into the early hours of Tuesday—but the first time they heard the full details was in court that Tuesday morning.[19]

At $35 million, the financial settlement fell far below the $1 billion the suit sought but, according to a news report that day, the money "seemed almost an afterthought" for many former residents. What mattered more was "long-overdue recognition of their suffering." The most significant part of the settlement, for many residents, was the promise of a formal apology from the premier. Patricia Seth explained that the apology would help bring closure. "I'm just elated to . . . not necessarily put the past at rest but put it on the back burner, because you can never forget something like that," she said. "We can move forward now, tell our stories. People believe us now."[20]

The settlement included other ways of acknowledging past suffering. It promised to place a commemorative plaque on the Huronia grounds. The buildings would be reopened for a number of days so former residents could visit in hopes of finding some closure and reminding them of details that might help them to prepare their compensation claims. Scholars would be given access to artifacts still on the site, and allowed to choose some for archives. The province would establish a registry for the hospital cemetery, where roughly two thousand children and adults were buried, more than fourteen hundred of them in graves without names. The registry was especially important, says Marilyn Dolmage. "The class action is about the survivors, but the survivors are honouring those that didn't survive."[21] Finally, the province agreed to scan electronically and deposit about sixty-five thousand documents related to the institution in the Archives of Ontario. As for the money, a point system would determine the amount an individual received, depending on the severity of the alleged abuses set out in the claim. The minimum payment would be $2,000; the maximum $42,000.[22]

In early December, just a few days after the court signed off on the settlement agreement, Premier Kathleen Wynne issued the apology. She did so in the legislative chamber, speaking directly to more than one

hundred Huronia, Rideau Regional, and Southwestern Ontario survivors, friends, family, and supporters who sat in the public gallery, and
to the "many others who couldn't make it" to the legislature that day.
"Today, Mr. Speaker, we take responsibility for the suffering of these
people and their families," the premier said. "I offer an apology to the
men, women and children of Ontario who were failed by a model of institutional care for people with developmental disabilities. We must look
in the eyes of those who have been affected, and those they leave behind,
and say: 'We are sorry.' As Premier, and on behalf of all the people of
Ontario, I am sorry for your pain, for your losses, and for the impact
that these experiences must have had on your faith in this province,
and in your government. I am sorry for what you and your loved ones
experienced, and for the pain you carry to this day."[23] The leaders of the
Conservative and New Democratic parties—parties that had, at various
times, governed the province and therefore also been responsible for the
institutions—issued apologies as well. Several former residents wept as
the apologies were delivered.

It was a touching, uplifting moment. I choked up when I watched the
premier's apology, and I cheered when I heard, less than two weeks later,
that the Rideau Regional and Southwestern suits had also been settled, for
a total of $32.7 million.[24] It felt like a vindication of my mother's struggle
over sending Bill away. I think she would have especially appreciated how
an editorial in the *Toronto Star* described the significance of the apology:
"An apology cannot change the past. But hopefully, Wynne's gesture will
help heal the hurt and allow Huronia's former residents to move on."[25]

Because Bill died in 1995, my family had no material interest in the
case. But seeing it settled mattered deeply, nonetheless.

———

Euphoria never lasts as long as we'd like it to, and after it passes the gritty
details still have to be worked out. And here, as in so many other parts
of the story of institution residents, some things fell short of what they
could—and should—have been.

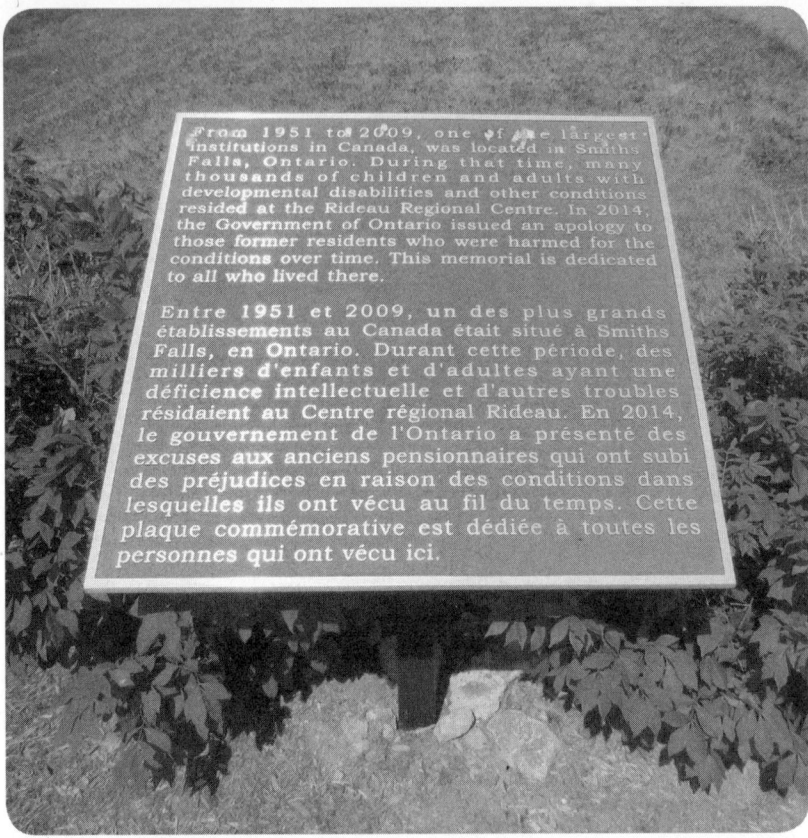

Plaque commemorating the Rideau Regional Centre (found at the Ontario
Provincial Police regional headquarters).

The plaques went up—one at each institution, more or less. In Smiths
Falls, the plaque is not actually on the grounds of the former hospital
school because the site has been sold to a private company. Instead, it's
at the Ontario Provincial Police regional headquarters, about half a
kilometre away. A sign on the road points to its location. The wording
was negotiated between the province and the lawyers running the class-
action suits. When all is said and done, the plaques are less than fulsome
in acknowledging the horrors of institutional life. The Huronia one
says: "From 1876 to 2009, many thousands of children and adults with
developmental disabilities and other conditions resided in the wards,

called 'cottages,' of this institution. In 2013, the government of Ontario issued an apology to the former residents for conditions over time." The ones at Rideau Regional and Southwestern Ontario say that the apologies went out in 2014 to "those former residents who were harmed by conditions over time," adding, "This memorial is dedicated to all who lived there."

The cemetery at Huronia has a new fence and new markers at the end of every row, despite concerns that the names on the row markers don't match the graves. The number of people buried is subject to dispute, and many were interred in unmarked graves or in graves signified only by numbers. A number of grave markers had been moved over the years. At one point someone took a bunch to use as patio stones at a nearby house, although the markers have since been returned.[26] A group of survivors and their allies known as Remember Every Name suspects that sewage pipes running through the graveyard may have disturbed about a hundred and fifty graves.[27] Leah Dolmage, Jim and Marilyn's daughter and one of the driving forces behind the Facebook group for Remember Every Name, says survivors wanted to play an active part in fixing the cemetery, but have been left feeling ignored and betrayed by the way the province has handled their concerns. She says the group is working on an alternate memorial that will do a better job of honouring the dead.[28]

Many former residents were able to get copies of their personal records from Huronia, Rideau Regional, or Southwestern Ontario, but the process was slow and uneven. As of the middle of 2014, two thousand people had applied for their files. The government had released 915, and was still working on another thousand or so. The government had also informed ninety former Huronia residents that their files could not be found.[29] It's hard to miss the irony here. Institution residents were, in many ways, non-persons — people whose civil rights had been stripped away, and whose presence had been erased from their homes and their families. And now, their institutional history has been erased, too.

The most heartbreaking fallout from the suits for Marie Slark, Patricia Smith, and Jim and Marilyn Dolmage was the process that determined how much compensation a former resident would receive. To claim amounts higher than the basic payout of $2,000, former residents had to fill out forms specifying incidents of non-consensual sex, injuries resulting from assault, or other abuse. This meant they not only had to revive some terrible memories, but they also had to recount them in detail in such a way as would meet the requirements of the settlement terms. That task was painfully difficult for many residents, and impossible for those who had very limited communication skills. Marilyn Dolmage says she was dismayed when she learned of this requirement: "Everything about the case was about neglect. The whole case was certified on the systemic issues: underfunding, understaffing and overcrowding leading to neglect. We were preparing to have a trial that was mostly about neglect but then we ended up with a settlement that wasn't."[30] The people whose injuries and suffering were caused by neglect received the lowest amount, as did those who were unable to prove that they had suffered both abuse and neglect or that they had not consented to sexual activity. The process left them feeling like they had been assaulted a second time. Jim Dolmage told me that roughly eight hundred people from all three institutions had their claims for compensation downgraded. In all, 3,500 claims were made and a total of 3,427 cheques were mailed, totalling just over $37.5 million.[31]

There have been some positive developments since the suits were settled, however.

One is that the survivors of other institutions have been emboldened to file class-action suits of their own. A suit covering eighty-eight hundred former residents from twelve of the smaller institutions for people with intellectual impairments, launched in 2015, was settled two years later for $36 million. A class-action suit alleging physical, emotional, and sexual abuse at the W. Ross Macdonald School for the Blind, in Brantford, was also settled, this one for $8 million, in the spring of 2017.[32] A new class-action suit, launched in 2017, accused the government of failing to eliminate lengthy wait lists for support services for adults with developmental disabilities who live in the community. The statement of claim alleges that, once an individual reaches the age of eighteen, the government "arbitrarily and unreasonably" cuts off supports that individual had access to as a child. "Adults may spend years on the . . . wait lists, requiring family members or other caregivers to provide the necessary services or supports, or going without such services," the statement of claim says. The Ontario budget released in March of 2018 proposed an extra $1.8 billion to help the eighteen thousand people then on the wait list.[33] An election that June ousted the Liberals. Premier Doug Ford's Conservatives are expected to make significant changes to disability support programs.

Leftover funds from the first three class-action suits have been granted to a range of art and theatre projects that enable former residents to tell their stories and let others know what life was like in the institution. A grant from the federal Social Sciences and Humanities Research Council helped fund Recounting Huronia, a participatory, arts-based research project that allows former residents to create a record of their own experiences. Kate Rossiter, an associate professor of health studies at the Brantford campus of Wilfrid Laurier University, is principal investigator, and the project also runs a speakers bureau, with Marie Slark as one of the speakers. Slark has said that her goal is to not only share her own story, but make people understand how others were treated in the institutions. "No amount of money could pay for what the government did," she said. "We need to have justice for people with disabilities."[34]

—

So many of the stories former institution residents tell are tales of deprivation, humiliation, or abuse of a sort that seems to be built into the institutional system itself. Several of the former Rideau Regional staff members I spoke to told similar tales. A woman who did a student placement there in the early 1980s said the atmosphere on her ward was always one of distress: screaming, manhandling, and frequent drug use to sedate people. A former staff member characterized the ward she worked on in the same decade as "extremely abusive." Staff members lied to families about what went on in the wards, she said, or pretended they didn't know how injuries occurred. She recalled one incident where a female resident startled a male employee on the night shift; he punched her in the eye. When a resident urinated in her bath, she recalls, a staff member held her head under the water. In another disturbing incident, a staff member dragged a woman, who wouldn't stay on the grass, along the pavement. This former staff member told me that when she was working on a ward for elderly residents some years later, she was appalled by the way some of her colleagues fed the residents. "They took the main meal, the dessert, and the drink, dumped it all into a bowl, and fed it to them as slop." Another former staff member recalled watching a male attendant chase down a boy who had stolen a bag of cookies from a locker on the ward. The boy wound up with a perforated eardrum. The supervisor brushed off the injury, saying the attendant was near retirement age and would be gone soon anyway.

For outsiders, and especially for families of former residents, systemic violence is a hard idea to grasp. A new book that draws on interviews done through the Recounting Huronia project offers some guidance in understanding the concept. Kate Rossiter and Jen Rinaldi, a legal studies professor at the University of Ontario Institute of Technology, note that reports of violence have emerged from a range of institutions in recent years: psychiatric facilities, residential schools, and retirement homes, as well as those for people with intellectual disabilities. "Common to all of these sites are two features. First, they are places ostensibly designed to provide care for people deemed vulnerable. Second, in each of these sites profound, and even sadistic, forms of violence have been inflicted on residents," the authors write.[35] The worst cases spark public outrage, but Rossiter and Rinaldi argue that these incidents are related to the routine, mundane forms of violence — daily acts of humiliation, degradation, neglect, punishment, and abuse — that are central to the operation of the institution. "We believe that practices of incarceration are in and of themselves violent, and necessarily produce further violence," they write. A number of conditions contribute to institutional violence: locating the facilities in rural areas where residents are socially isolated; operating them under conditions of austerity or for profit; seeing their mandate as reforming people in their care; housing people who are socially devalued or despised; and giving staff members a high degree of control over the residents. "I have yet to find an institution that meets these criteria that isn't violent," Rossiter told a CBC interviewer in 2018.[36]

Rossiter and Rinaldi say institutional violence occurs along a spectrum. At one end is "cold violence," or the dozens of large and small indignities of daily life on the inside. "Cold violence" is characterized by a denial of individual choice, privacy, and dignity, and by the use of shame-inducing rituals, like post-shower penis inspections for uncircumcised boys at Huronia. "Warm violence" refers to the way the institution handles transgressions—slapping, spanking, solitary confinement in so-called side rooms, restraints, and tranquilizers. The goal, ostensibly, is to correct what the institution defines as "bad behaviour," and encourage compliance with the rules. At the other end of the spectrum is "hot violence"—rape and other sexual abuse, torture, and acts of sheer cruelty with the sole purpose of gratifying the person inflicting the pain. It's the kind of violence that is likely to attract media attention or, in some cases, lead to criminal charges.

It was tempting for the people running the institutions to see the stories of the representative plaintiffs as exceptions: regrettable but isolated incidents in institutional life. In its statement of defence against the Huronia suit, for example, the government denied that systemic abuse, mistreatment, or assault occurred at the institution and maintained that, if incidents did occur, "the Crown was not made aware of these allegations at the relevant time."[37] When incidents of what Rossiter and Rinaldi would call "hot violence" came to the attention of provincial authorities, the government argued, they investigated and handled the cases in an appropriate way. And that's partly true. In 1979, for example, opposition politicians asked the minister of community and social services, Keith Norton, for a report on the extent of abuse by staff in the institutions. Norton replied that his ministry had undertaken twelve separate investigations of twenty-eight incidents of abuse or suspected

abuse at the facilities in 1978. Eighteen of the incidents were cases where
a staff member hit a resident. Others included encouraging residents to
hit each other, taping a resident's mouth shut, burning residents with a
cigarette, having sex with residents, pouring cold water on a resident, and
stepping on and crushing a resident's penis. Norton added that three of
the twelve employees implicated were dismissed. Two were ordered on
unpaid leave. Four got written warnings, and three of them were cleared
because of insufficient evidence. The minister noted that eleven of the
thirteen incidents reported at Rideau Regional were attributed to a single
employee.[38] The reassuring message the minister sought to convey was
that the authorities would respond rigorously and effectively when they
discovered a bad apple on the staff. What's missing, however, is why this
kind of violence happened in the first place, or how one employee got
away with abuse for so long.

Investigations happened only when an incident was formally reported,
and many residents did not, could not, or would not report them. Others
told ward staff about incidents but were ignored, not believed, threatened,
or told to just let things lie. Reports of staff abuse, when they did appear,
often came from other staff members or from students doing internships.
It's certain, therefore, that many incidents simply went unreported or
uninvestigated.

A good deal of evidence about institutional violence is in the Archives
of Ontario, if you have the stomach to go through it.[39] The set of electronic records created as part of the class-action suit settlements includes
hundreds of documents — serious occurrence reports; contentious issue
reports; incident memos; resident incident, accident, and injury reports;
medication or treatment error reports, and more — that make for difficult reading. The forms were filled out by employees, which means they
give the staff member's interpretation of an incident, not the resident's,
and the volume of reports increased over the years as the reporting requirements got more and more strict. Reports from Rideau Regional,
dating from the 1970s to the 2000s, show a remarkable range of staff

misbehaviour, ranging from the inappropriate to the potentially criminal: a staff member burned a resident on the back with a cigarette; students on a work placement reported physical and verbal abuse of residents by staff; a staff member reported that she had slapped a resident (a cleaner witnessed the slap, which may have been the reason the staff member reported it); a student reported a staff member abusing a male resident; a staff member reported that another staff member abused at least two residents; a staff member gave medication in an "inappropriate and dangerous manner"; three staff members failed to provide CPR to a dying resident; a housekeeper was accused of having sex with a resident; a different housekeeper was found with a female resident in a locked room in the basement; a staff member delivered the wrong meals, giving regular food to people who needed pureed food to prevent choking; a male staff member assaulted a female resident, causing bruising and internal bleeding that required hospital care; eight residents told a staff member that another staff member had abused them over three years; a staff member showed up for work drunk; a staff member routinely hit residents with a broomstick.

The institutions had detailed policies on using physical holds and mechanical restraints, which were reviewed and updated frequently. The policies said restraints should be used to protect individuals from harming themselves or others, not as a punishment or to suit staff convenience. The people who worked with residents were to be certified annually in how to use them, and the length of time a resident spent in restraints was to be strictly limited and monitored. Nonetheless, injuries happened. A particularly tragic incident in the 1990s involved a woman in her twenties who had been at Smiths Falls for nine years. One day in April 1993, according to the report, the woman became self-abusive and then assaulted her counsellor, who put her in a restraint hold. The resident quieted down, but moved from one couch to another. A supervisor later saw her on the floor and asked her to get on the couch, which she did with the help of this supervisor. But she slid off the couch again and lay on the floor, not moving. The staff thought this was "attention-seeking" behaviour. It was not—she had a dislocated vertebra in her neck. Airlifted to a hospital in Kingston, she died there ten days later. Had she lived, she would have been paralyzed.

A considerable amount of violent behaviour originated with the residents themselves. Given the atmosphere in which they lived and the fact that for many acting out was a way to communicate, this is not surprising. Some residents were genuinely dangerous to others. The province wrote and rewrote policies aimed at showing staff how to keep potentially dangerous residents, and the others, safe. In some cases, though, some residents who had been ordered isolated ended up hurting others anyway. For instance, a man with a developmental disability who had been accused of forcible confinement and assault of two children in another town ended up at the Rideau Regional Centre in December 2002. He was meant to stay at the facility until a better living situation could be arranged. Two months later, two women residents reported, separately, that the man had sexually assaulted them. The Ontario Provincial Police decided not to lay charges because the women were legally incompetent witnesses. Eventually the man was charged with three counts of uttering death threats, one of assault, and one of breaching a court order. In 1984, one of Bill's fellow Dundas ward residents was referred to the Queen's University sexual offenders clinic after a series of sexually aggressive incidents against other men.

Violent outbursts could be terrifying—and dangerous—for both the staff and other residents. In one case, a male resident charged across a room to attack a woman. The ward staff called for help, and the man was put into a five-point restraint and dosed with Haldol, a powerful anti-psychotic. Over the next seventy minutes he struggled so much he "bounced his bed across the ward" and other residents had to be moved, according to the incident report. Eventually, the man calmed down. In another incident, a staff member reported that he broke up a fight and got the aggressor to calm down. About fifteen minutes later, the resident began "yelling and hitting the coffee table" then threw his coffee cup and smashed it. The staff member said he took the resident into the office, gave him Haldol, and told him to go and lie down. "[He] then attacked me," the staff member reported. "He kicked, I blocked it. He then threw a punch. I blocked and ducked, it glanced off the left side of my head above my ear." A "staff alert" brought extra help to the ward. The resident was put in restraints.

Many, many accident and injury reports on file in the archives list the cause as unknown. This goes for bite marks, bruises, missing teeth, cuts, and broken bones. Some reports cite staff carelessness that led to injuries — leaving residents unattended on a dressing table, for example, or neglecting to buckle them into their wheelchairs. In one case, a staff member left a resident alone in the shower to go and help restrain another resident. The one in the shower drank the shampoo. In another, a resident left alone tried to eat Ajax cleanser. But the number of unexplained injuries, in an institution where people were to receive round-the-clock care and supervision, is beyond disturbing.

The people working at the institutions did so under stressful conditions, and some dealt with their stress by using alcohol or drugs while on duty. Some, as the archived documents show, turned on each other. A man was reported for the sexual harassment of two colleagues after he brought pornography to work and shared it around. Another man made death threats against three female colleagues. A staff member threw a knife at a colleague. A male manager harassed and assaulted a female employee. An employee made eight allegations against several colleagues, including assault of residents, that turned out to be unfounded. Apparently this particular employee had a history of making threats against other staff.

It's hard to square the documents I read in that little glassed-in room at the archives with the staff members I met at Rideau Regional when Bill was an adult. They took their jobs seriously, formed genuine relationships with Bill, showed extreme patience supervising him as he did his chores, and shared the joy of accomplishment when he picked up a new skill. The families who sued to keep the institutions open also had a high regard for the staff. They respected their professionalism, their knowledge, and their care. They recognized the bonds the staff had forged with relatives on the inside, and they were loath to deprive their relatives of the people who mattered to them deeply. It must have been especially difficult for these caring and concerned employees to work with others they knew — or suspected — had abused residents or co-workers. As one former staff member told me, "Sometimes I didn't like the people I worked with, but I always liked the people I worked for."

Some former staff members were deeply hurt by the wording of the commemorative plaque. They felt it painted them all — those who worked there in the harshest years before the Williston report, and those whose careers covered the later, far better years — with the same brush. They tried to start an online petition to have it changed.[40] And while many former staff members were glad to see the institutions close and applauded the class-action suits, others did not. They worried about whether the former residents would get adequate care in the community. Some of them also worried about being stigmatized as burnout cases or abusers, which might make it hard for them to find other work.

I understand their concerns. The problem was not a matter of lumping the good staff in with the bad, however, but the institutional system itself. As governments since the 1970s have acknowledged, and as a growing number of scholars have shown,[41] it was a failed model of care for people like my brother. But, like the crooked roulette wheel gamblers play even when they know it's crooked, that system was the only game in town for generations of families, including my own.

—

In my search to recapture my brother's life, I found no record of the first time someone hit Bill at Smiths Falls. But I did find a record of the last; it's in his medical file. On April 14, 1995, three weeks before he died, a fellow resident hit him while he was sitting in the lounge in the institution's hospital unit. Upset, he went to find the nurse. "No injuries noted," the nursing notes say.

Chapter 12

"WE NEVER SEEM TO **FIND TIME** TO **TALK ABOUT BILL**"

One chilly afternoon in early December 1985, I came home from work to find a bulky letter in my mailbox. I recognized the handwriting on the envelope immediately: it was my mother's. I was living in Kingston then, having brought my American family north the summer before, and we were due to visit Mom and Dad over the holidays, so the sight of a fat letter from Mom was puzzling. I was even more puzzled when I opened the envelope. Inside was a photocopy of a long, handwritten letter in my mother's even and artful script. In blue ink at the top of the first page, she had added a note saying she'd sent copies to my sister, Mary, and brother Bob, too.

"This morning I had a dream about Billy and wakened with such a feeling of guilt regarding him that I couldn't go back to sleep," Mom wrote. "I got up, went into the den and had myself a weep and thought of how divorced he is from our and your lives—and he is our child just as you are." I immediately sat down to read the rest. When I finished, I was still puzzled. Though the letter itself came as a surprise, the stories she recited in it—Bill throwing up on the barber, the mountains of laundry, the psychiatrist who warned Dad that he shouldn't let Mom bring the baby home, the maids who didn't quite work out, Bill throwing up on Mary's dress—were old news. We had heard them often over the years. The only genuinely new detail was Dad's telephone call to the superintendent at Smiths Falls to ask about admitting a newborn directly from the hospital where he was born. I knew Dad had been the driving force behind sending Bill to Smiths Falls, but I had not realized Dad had tried to send him there so quickly.

The real surprise in the letter was this: "I realize you don't remember him because it was so long ago that he left, so I decided to tell you the story of Bill and our lives." Of course we remembered Bill. Mary and I both had memories of Bill at home, though Bob was too young for that. We had pictures of him in the family photo albums, taken when he was at home and after he left. We visited him every month throughout our childhoods, so often that we probably could have found our way to the hospital school blindfolded. Not remember Bill? What a strange thing to say!

And then, near the end of the letter, she wrote: "I have gone on at great length but when you are home we never seem to find time to talk about Bill." I felt stung. I kept track of her visits and asked her about him after every one. I sent him birthday and Christmas cards. I offered to go with Mom to Smiths Falls whenever I was in Ottawa, even though I knew she would say no. Not talk about Bill—what on earth did she mean? It took me years to figure that one out, but I think I finally understand. What we did not talk about was the pain and guilt she felt about sending Bill away—and keeping him away—from our family. But, truth be told, she was too conflicted to talk with us about her feelings and too tightly wound to want to hear about our feelings either: especially if, as she feared, we might have a different opinion about what happened to Bill. She saw Bill as her personal cross to bear, and hers alone. Any fears or regrets or anger the rest felt would only add to her burden. Mary and Bob and I knew how deep her guilt ran; after all, we had grown up with it. And we had all decided, on our own and without talking to each other, not to press her about it. But that doesn't mean we didn't see it, or think about what Bill meant to our family.

Bill upended the life Mom and Dad had worked so carefully to create. Nowadays, we'd dismiss as ridiculous Aunt Ella's attempt to blame Bill's disability on "tainted blood" in my mother's family. In those days, though, the shame that came with intellectual disability was palpable, and Ella's comment cut deep. And the chaos Bill brought to our household when he began throwing up at eighteen months pushed Mom to the limit. She kept the family together for a while, but in the end she was the one who filled out the paperwork to admit Bill to the hospital school at Smiths Falls. She was the one who took him to the pediatrician for the note certifying him as "mentally defective." She was the one who packed his things.

I understand why my parents decided to send Bill to the hospital school. I understand that they worried about his future, as well as theirs and ours. Activists for children with disabilities were beginning to push for community schools and, eventually, for integration into the regular school system. They would succeed, but that was still years in the future. And my parents weren't activists. They could not imagine confronting authority or turning us into a poster family for children with intellectual disabilities. If the people they respected told them that sending Bill away was the right thing to do, that was all they had to hear.

The fact the institution was in the hands of doctors and nurses would have made that choice easier for my parents. These were colleagues, people who spoke the same professional language as my parents and shared the same professional values. The starched nurses' uniforms, which other parents might have found odd or maybe even intimidating, would have felt reassuring to my parents. The "hospital" part of the hospital school, with its promise of cleanliness and efficient routines, would have given them confidence. The "school" part was a frill, as they saw it, a nice chance for Bill to learn what he could or at least to give some structure to his days. They had no expectations that he would learn much, and the more he failed to learn the more convinced they became that they had made the right choice. They believed that Bill would never be able to survive in the "real" world, and would remain a child even if he beat the odds and survived into adulthood.

So many of the choices we make in life are complex. My parents also knew their own lives would be easier without Bill in the house. They wanted a fourth child, and were ready to take on the extra work that would come with that child. The problem was that they didn't get the child they wanted; they got a "mongoloid." The previous generation kept children with intellectual disabilities a secret out of shame or embarrassment. My parents felt lucky that they could make the more modern choice of sending Bill to live with what the experts euphemistically called "his own kind" but still keep in touch with him. The fact *we*, his brother and sisters, were his own kind was irrelevant. Disability trumped family.

As they got older and Mom's health declined, or when they read about the problems other aging parents encountered trying to find homes or care for their adult children with intellectual impairments, they would smile at each other with relief at how wise they had been to send Bill away. But the speed with which they made that choice, the fact they looked into sending their newborn straight to Smiths Falls without ever bringing him home, still surprises me. In my darkest moments I wonder what would have happened if Dad had succeeded in transferring Bill directly to the institution. It's possible that he would have tried to convince Mom to come up with a convenient lie that would keep Bill's existence a secret, perhaps even from the rest of us.

Throughout all those years Bill lived away from us, and even after he died, my parents never edited the family mantra. Until the end of their lives, it was "sending Bill away was the best thing we could have done *for him*," not "sending Bill away was the best thing we could have done *for us*." Of course it wasn't that clean or that simple.

I really don't know what prompted Mom to write that long *cri de coeur* to Mary, Bob, and me back in 1985. Perhaps she'd had another run-in with the institution about getting Bill off the anti-seizure drug he had been taking for far too long. Perhaps this was when she learned that he had chronic hepatitis B. Perhaps she and Dad had argued, again, over bringing Bill home for Christmas. Or maybe she was simply feeling wistful as Christmas approached and the rest of us got ready to come home for the holidays. It did, however, allow her to express some of her sorrow and pain and guilt. But only some. She told the safe stories — small incidents with no bad guys, stories about two parents trying to do what was best for all their children. Even the arguments she and Dad had about bringing Bill home for visits ended on a positive note. She might have regrets, but she accepted Dad's view. The letter concluded with a final, wistful paragraph: "I hope I have covered all the bases and made you more aware of your younger brother. He knows me when I go up but I'm sure the concept of 'mother' is beyond him — I'm just the nice lady who takes him to lunch. *Finis*." This sounded rehearsed when I first read it. Thirty years later, it still does. But I think it was the only way she knew how to confront the fact that, by sending Bill away from our family, our family had become irrelevant to Bill.

Mom's letter, however, was a record, even if an imperfect one, of how she felt about Bill. What Bill meant to Dad is far more difficult to pin down. Behind his kind and genuinely warm exterior, Dad was never good at sorting out his feelings and even less accomplished at discussing them. He would never dream of confiding any worries or uncertainties he might have felt about Bill to his other children or his sons-in-law. That would have been a sign of weakness, and weakness was forbidden. The only written record he left of Bill is in the quirky family history — it's part genealogy and part personal essays by various family members — compiled by his cousin Elizabeth Stuart. Dad wrote:

> Our youngest child, Billy, was born on Sept. 6, 1956.
> He was a lovable, friendly Down's Syndrome youngster.
> Eventually he lived at the Smiths Falls Hospital School
> where he was tenderly cared for. We saw him often and he
> loved his mother. Unfortunately, he developed Hepatitis
> and died in May, 1995. We always wondered if we had
> done the right thing in sending him to Smiths Falls,
> but any doubts we ever had were dispelled during his
> last illness when the care and compassion that he — and

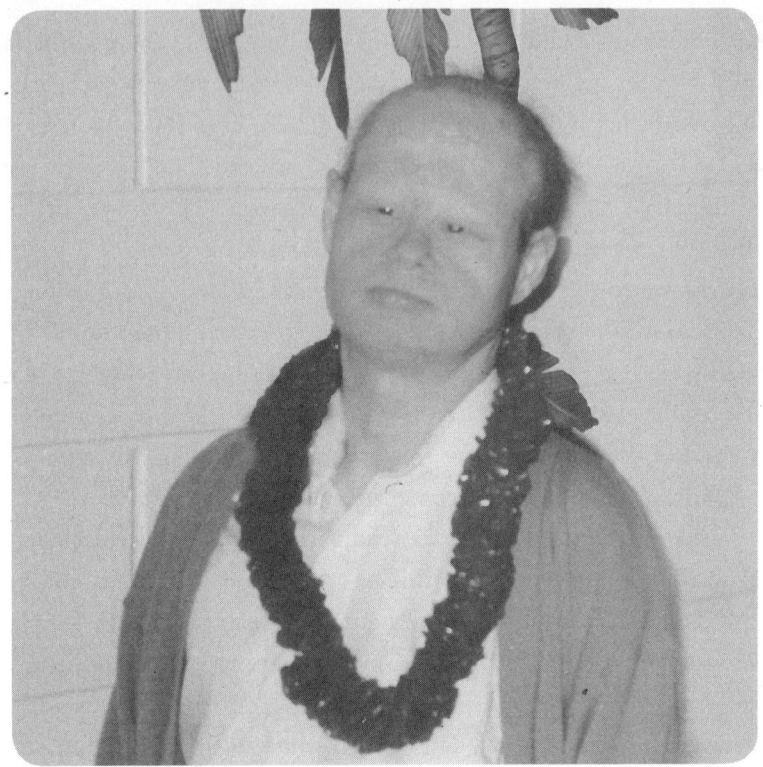

Years of institutional living are inscribed on Bill's face in this
photo taken at a Hawaiian-themed party in the early 1990s.

we—received convinced us he had been well taken care
of. His funeral, which was held at the school among his
peers, was a very moving experience that all of us will
remember.[1]

This was the closest Dad ever came to admitting *any* doubts about
whether his decision to commit Bill to the institution was the right call.
But, after opening that door by the tiniest crack, he slams it shut immediately. And his words conceal so much more than they reveal. Bill
"eventually" moved to Smiths Falls ("eventually" was at the age of two
and a half). Bill "unfortunately" came down with hepatitis (the word

suggests it was an accident, and yet I know he blamed the medical staff). Bill was "tenderly" cared for at Rideau Regional (how does that explain the bruises and scars he saw on every visit?). The institution treated Bill and the family with "care and compassion" when he died (does mailing them a consent-to-treatment form for their dead son show either?). In short, Dad's comment suggests, no harm, no foul.

Surely it wasn't that simple. Especially for Dad.

Dad knew what it was like to have your father turn his back on you. His own father had walked out on his family when Dad was in his late teens. Dad never forgave him. His essay in the family history is close to fifteen hundred words long and contains lots of memories of his grandfather, his childhood, his early days in medicine, trips he took with Mom, and other highlights of his life. Bert gets two lines. After identifying him as his father and reporting that he ran the general store in Vernon, Ontario, Dad doesn't mention Bert again. Two lines—that's it. I don't know if Mom ever met Bert; probably not. As children we didn't even know we *had* a living grandfather, much less a grandfather who lived within easy driving distance. I didn't see a picture of him until I was an adult.

As far as I know, Dad saw Bert twice during my lifetime. The first time was when Bert showed up ill at the hospital emergency room in the early 1950s. Dad, who was in the building checking on his own patients, got a call from an ER doctor asking him to come down. Dad did, probably because it would have looked bad to refuse. The second time was at Bert's funeral.

Clearly, being abandoned by his father hurt my father deeply. So I have to wonder whether Dad, the abandoned son, had any second thoughts about sending his own son away from the family. Did he even see the irony? I wish I knew.

As Dad neared the end of his life, Bert began to turn up now and then in the stories he told us about his childhood. Bert loved cars and taught Dad how to drive long before he was old enough to get his licence. Bert was especially proud of a car with a newfangled device, an electric cigarette lighter. After using it one day, Bert shook it like a match and tossed it out the car window. He screeched to a halt and searched for it, but the lighter was gone for good. Bert took the family on road trips up north to see the Dionne quintuplets, and southwest to see Niagara Falls. Like the few wartime stories he would share with us, these were happy stories, or funny ones. They hid the scars.

Dad died of cancer in 2011. His last six weeks were at a hospice that was a short walk from my house. The hours we spent there every day were among the most intimate we shared. One day when Dad was very near the end, dozy from the morphine and not in much pain, my husband mentioned how much he'd loved going to the Horn & Hardart Automat when he was growing up in New York. Dad perked up. He loved that place too, he said. Then he turned to me.

"Say," he said, "do you remember when we all went to the Automat?"

It took me a moment to reply, not because I didn't remember but because I knew it had never happened. "Um, I'm not sure, Dad," I said. "Remind me."

He launched into a story about how Bert drove us all—including Vinny, Rosemary, and Madeline—to the Horn & Hardart Automat for pie. He described how we dropped coins in slots, opened the little doors, and took out the slices. The pie was delicious, he added with a smile. Then a confused look crept over his face. He realized that the story didn't hold up. He knew I had never met Bert, and Bert had been dead for fifteen years before my daughters were born. Dad waved his hand vaguely, as if to wipe away the errant memory, and fell silent. But I was struck by the sweetness of a fantasy that repaired his broken family with a nice slice of pie.

—

Mary, Bob, and I grew up in a family that was fractured in a way that was invisible to most people, even at times to us. Had Bill died as an infant —and he came close a couple of times, including that horrible bout of pneumonia when he was a toddler—our friends and family would have rallied to see us through our grief at his death. It would have been terrible for everyone, and we would have tried over the years to keep our memories of Bill alive. But it would have been a clean and sharp-edged loss. It would have left a scar, but with time the scar would have faded.

Sending Bill to the hospital school was a different kind of break, less sharp but no less deep. On the one day a month when we visited him, he was as solid and real as the rest of us, and our family was whole. Otherwise, Bill was a phantom—a part of the family but apart from the family. And those visiting days could be wrenching. We welcomed him back into the family and said goodbye again over a few hours, behaving as though this was a perfectly normal thing for a family to do and smiling in cheerful solidarity with our parents. The scars his departure left never healed; each visit tore them open again until eventually, one by one, we simply stopped going. With every day that we did not visit him, he faded more and more from our lives. No one asked about him. Many of our friends and acquaintances didn't even know he existed. He was invisible.

The fact Mary, Bob, and I can't remember the day our parents took him away says something, I think, though I wish I knew what. It's possible we were so well prepared for his departure that we simply accepted it, and didn't see it as a memorable event. It's equally possible that we were so confused or traumatized by it that we wiped it from our memories. Or perhaps our parents told us he was going away for a little while, and we realized only as the days turned into weeks and the weeks into months that he wasn't coming back. I have no idea, and no way of finding out.

What we did know, from just about the moment he was born, was that something was wrong with Bill. Something bad—really, really bad. We were all too young to understand what a congenital condition like Down syndrome was, but we knew that this bad thing Bill had, whatever it was, meant *he* was bad—so bad, in fact, that he had to be ejected from the family. The lesson I took from this as a child was that if one of us could be sent away for being bad, then the rest of us had better make darn sure we were "good." Otherwise, we might be next.

Love was never an issue in our family but suddenly, with Bill's departure, acceptance was. And so was trust.

These days, a family like ours would go for counselling to help cope with the loss of a child. For us, that was unthinkable. Dad used to say, only half-jokingly, that psychiatrists were crazy, so you'd really have to be crazy to go see one. He didn't have much time for psychologists either. Again only half-jokingly, he used to say that PhD stood for "Phony Doctor." Bad jokes aside, I think he would have been embarrassed to go for counselling alone or with the rest of us, worried that people would gossip, and probably afraid that if the news leaked out that he needed mental health help it might drive away patients. His livelihood depended on people believing he was strong and stable and trustworthy, as well as warm and kind. Above all, though, I think he was too proud to seek help, or to let anyone see his pain. On this or any other loss. He did what he always did when something bad happened in his life: he tamped down his feelings and carried on, and he expected the rest of us would all do the same.

As we grew older and understood more about the reasons our parents did what they did, the fear of being sent away like Bill faded. But the lesson that family acceptance depended on being "good" lasted a long, long time. We all developed, in one way or another, a habit of trying far harder than we should to please our parents, to avoid displeasing them, or to fly under their radar when we wanted to do something we knew they wouldn't like. All kids do this to some degree; I think our reaction was more extreme. We all felt, one way or another, that we had to measure up to the perfect family Dad and Mom envisioned, and we knew that somehow we never could. Each of us has admitted to feeling like an outsider in our own family. All of us had to leave home — actually, leave the country — to become the adults we wanted to be.

The lack of trust inside our family showed up in different ways. Bob says he grew up fearful of asking for things directly, "in case the answer was, 'No, I don't like you, and I want to send you far, far, away.'" He hung back, hoped people would see what he wanted, and was disappointed when they didn't. Bob says has always been afraid of rejection and has dealt with depression all his life. Mary became the disciplinarian, keeping Bob and me in line. But I think there was a protective impulse at work here too, even if none of us recognized it: keeping order was a way of keeping us safe. I took a more confrontational approach. Mom and Dad often wanted us to do things "for our own good." I never trusted that phrase. It was too close to the way they talked about how sending Bill away was for *his* own good. My first instinct was to suspect that whatever it was they wanted me to do — take this course in high school rather than that course, go to this university rather than to that university, date a doctor rather than become a doctor — suited their interests more than mine. My second instinct was to resist, to do everything but what they wanted. I fought them on just about everything, large or small. In some ways that made me a stronger person. But it took me years to figure out when to let the small stuff slide, to trust that they could appreciate me for my differences even if they didn't understand what those differences were.

Perhaps the biggest impact our strange, fractured childhood had on us as adults showed up when it was time to consider having children of our own. As Mom feared, Mary developed an aversion to small children, especially babies. She would never hurt one, of course, but she doesn't like being around them, and she has no desire to cuddle them or even touch them. If someone hands her a baby she reacts as if she's been handed a grenade, waiting for it to explode in gross or disgusting ways. Her dislike of children began early, when she was still more or less a child herself, and how much of it can be traced directly to Bill is impossible to say. She knew, as a young adult, that motherhood was not for her and had herself sterilized when she was in her late twenties, before she met her husband, Richard. She has never regretted that decision.

Bob and I wanted children, and the spectre of Down syndrome loomed over that decision for both of us.

Given that the chances of giving birth to a child with Down syndrome rise after the mother hits the age of thirty-five — and that Mom had Bill when she was thirty-six — I decided long before I met the man I would marry that I would have my children before I was thirty, just to be on the safe side. If I didn't have a partner by that age, I figured (probably foolishly) that I would go ahead on my own. Happily, I met Vinny. Mom and Dad were the first people I called when I got pregnant. They congratulated us, and then Mom immediately told me to get genetic counselling and ask about a prenatal test known as amniocentesis to check for Down syndrome. If the fetus had Down syndrome, she said, I could get rid of it early. I hung up the phone thinking how bizarre it was to talk to my mother about abortion before I'd even told my friends I was pregnant. I am sure she knew, on some level, that this was a horrible thing to say to me, but she couldn't help herself. And I wasn't surprised by her reaction. I did talk to my doctor about this test, and he ruled it out: given my age—I was twenty-seven—the odds that the test would cause a miscarriage were far higher than the possibility of the fetus having Down syndrome. That was fine with me, but Mom fretted and worried all the way through that pregnancy and the next one two years later. Mom was dead before Bob's daughter, Eve, was born. No doubt she would have fretted even more about that pregnancy, given that Bob and his wife were older when they became parents than I was. Like me, my brother and his wife sought genetic counselling. They went ahead with amniocentesis.

Had I learned that I was carrying a fetus with Down syndrome, I would have had an abortion. Without question. Bob would have made the same decision. We did not want to go through the agonies Mom had gone through over Bill, and I worried that another child with Down syndrome in the family might, quite literally, kill my mother. I don't think I'd make the same decision today, though I'd go to the barricades to protect a woman's right to make her own choice. As of this writing, a number of US states—among them North Dakota, Ohio, Indiana, Louisiana, and Pennsylvania—are using the availability of new and non-invasive prenatal tests as a pretext for drawing up legislation to prevent women from aborting a fetus with Down syndrome. Columnist George F. Will even used Nazi-era words like *genocide* and *final solution* to describe termination of fetuses with the condition.[2] Like Michael Berube, the author of two books about raising a son who has Down syndrome, I see the cynicism behind these laws. "Don't try to tell us that the lawmakers behind HB 2050 [the Pennsylvania bill] care about the lives of people with Down syndrome," Berube writes. "This bill's supporters are overwhelmingly hard-right conservatives who have voted against *every kind of support* our Jamie needs—from early intervention programs, to inclusive education, to Medicaid." If they really cared about people with Down syndrome they'd push for better supports. "Instead, they're using Down syndrome as an excuse to roll back reproductive rights—and to divide pro-life and pro-choice families of people with Down syndrome."[3]

When our daughter Madeline called to tell us she was pregnant, that phone call with my mother came back to me. I know Madeline worried about Down syndrome, too. After all, Mom's grief and anxiety about Bill was a feature of her childhood, as it had been of mine. I hope she understood that Vinny and I were thrilled for her and her husband, and supported them fully as they became parents, and that we would love their children unconditionally, joyfully, and completely.

—

Mary, Bob, and I have all gone on to live full and rich lives. Mom and Dad did too, in love with each other and embracing life until the end. The tragic figure in our family story was Bill. People with Down syndrome have the same needs as everyone else: a home, an education, a chance to do meaningful work, and the love of family and friends. Bill's life came up short in almost every area. He grew up in a closed, cramped, crowded, impersonal, rigid, noisy, and sometimes violent environment, in a hospital school that was more warehouse than either hospital or school. He was certainly neglected during his childhood at Rideau Regional and, based on the experiences of other former institution residents, he was probably abused. His education, such as it was, got him nowhere. He did not get the speech therapy that might have helped him learn how to speak. He did not get the one-on-one training that might have taught him how to count or read. He did not get the psychological counselling or the appropriate therapy that might have eased his obsessive-compulsive tendencies. He spent nine years, almost one-quarter of his life, on a daily barbiturate because of a single seizure and most of the final year of his life on carbamazepine, a drug with toxic side effects. It's true that the institution became more humane in his adult years, and that Transition House C was, in many ways, a happy place for him to live. But he lost far more as a child and teenager than he could ever get back as an adult. And then he died of a disease he contracted simply because he lived in the institution. Had he not contracted hepatitis B, he'd be in his early sixties today. Instead, his life was over at thirty-eight.

Pretty well every item on the long, sad list of damages set out in the class-action suits against the province applied in Bill's case. The biggest loss he suffered, however, was love. Dad wrote that the people who took care of Bill did so tenderly, and I'm sure many did. But they worked for the institution, not for Bill. Their job was to take care of Bill's basic needs, get him to comply with the rules and routines of the institution, and make sure he didn't cause problems for other residents or staff. The

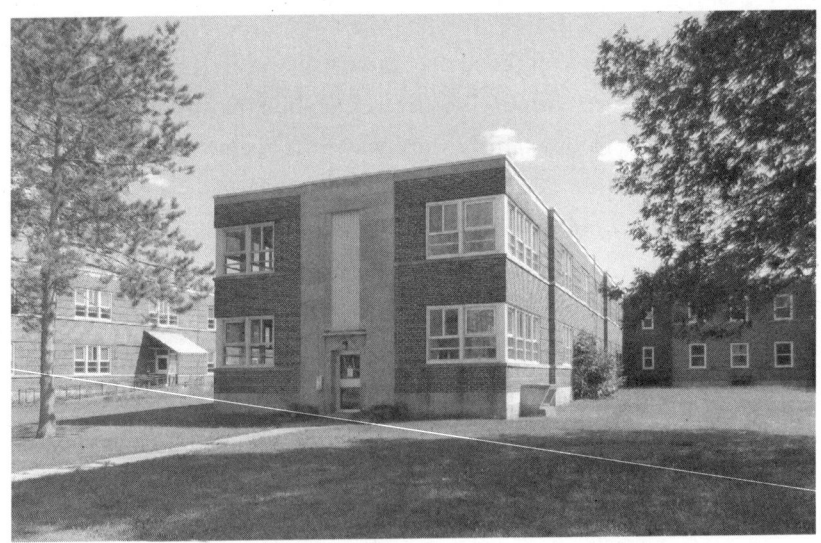

The bland facade of this typical ward block at Rideau Regional shows no hint of what life was like on the inside for thousands of people like Bill.

counsellor assigned as his primary caretaker would work with him for a few months or a year, or maybe two, and then move on. Several of the former staff members I talked to described the people in their care as "like family." I believe them when they say they felt genuine affection for them, and I know some stayed in touch with former clients long after the institution closed. When their shifts were over, though, they went home to their own families. When they were reassigned, they left Bill behind. When they left Rideau Regional for a new job, they disappeared from Bill's life. When Bill moved to a new ward, he left them behind. It didn't matter if he became emotionally attached to this counsellor or that one; they all disappeared from his daily life. Just like his sisters and brother. Just like his parents.

In a book I used to read to my own children, Robert Munsch captured the essence of unconditional family love: the mother rocking her sleeping child and singing, "I'll love you forever, I'll like you for always, as long as I'm living my baby you'll be."[4] That kind of love was an alien concept for Bill. No one was in his corner day by day and year by year. He had no one to make him feel special, or safe, or valued, or important, or unique: no one he could rely on for a hug regardless of whether he succeeded or failed, or was happy or sad or lonely or overwhelmed. Without a doubt he knew Mom loved him, and he loved her, but they saw each other once a month. The rest of the time she simply wasn't there.

If unconditional love was missing from his life, so was the capacity to make decisions about how to live. As a child and teenager he had no control over where or when he would move within the institution — no choice in which ward he lived in, or who would sleep in the beds next to him, or when he would get up or go to bed, or how he would spend his days. Even after the big wards were broken up into family-style units, the institution chose the people who would constitute his so-called family. Not Bill. When residents began to move away to group homes or other living arrangements, his institutional family began to disappear one by one. His social world, such as it was, got smaller and smaller. His life was one long series of breakups.

No wonder he resisted change so fiercely. No wonder he resorted to hair pulling or wall tapping or hiding food in his underwear drawer if it made him feel he had some control.

It didn't have to be that way. Contrast Bill's life with that of McGill professor David Wright's sister Susan, born just eleven years later in another city in the same province. Faced with the same choice as my parents — home or institution — David and Susan's parents chose home. This was not an easy choice, Wright recalls, but his parents were committed to making Susan's life the best it could be.

> The subsequent years were filled with battles that, only in retrospect, were such a reflection of the 1970s: the struggle to have my sister entered in kindergarten in the public school across the street, which my parents achieved, only to have her ultimately assigned to a series of separate schools in the mid-size, south-western Ontario city in which we had settled; convincing employers that she could work as a teenage employee in the private sector, a dream for my sister made possible by a compassionate manager at the local McDonald's restaurant; battles with the local community college to have her register in a course to learn how to read, despite their insistence that the course was not right for her "type," and that her presence would embarrass other students.[5]

With help and support from her family and from various agencies in the community, Susan built a life. She rented an apartment. She married a man who had spent forty years inside one of the Ontario institutions. "Susan continues, as an adult in her 40s, to live in what advocates refer to as a 'supported independent living' arrangement — in reality a modest two-bedroom apartment — with her husband," Wright notes. "Their life is rich and loving, a situation of complementary abilities, with continued support from my family and some help provided by local welfare agencies." Susan and her husband work. They bowl. They're ushers at church. They like to watch wrestling videos. They eat out at Swiss Chalet. Susan never learned to read, Wright says, but developed remarkable social skills "to the extent that she and her husband are well known and admired in the neighbourhood." The people who work in the local pharmacy, the grocery store, and other shops know them and go out of their way to support their desire "to live their lives independently and with dignity."[6]

Life for the current generation of young adults with Down syndrome is even more removed from my brother's experience, or Susan's. Ted Holmes of Kingston, Ontario, says that when his son Evan was born in 1992, no one even raised the idea of sending him into care. Evan went to the local public elementary and high schools. He always had the help of an educational aide. He stayed in high school until he aged out of the system at twenty-one. He spends his days at the H'art Centre, which runs arts programs for adults with developmental disabilities. Ted Holmes worked as a student at Huronia and for a year as a counsellor at Rideau Regional, so he is more familiar than most with what institutional life was like for children with Down syndrome. Evan has a much better life. When Evan needed open-heart surgery at six months, there was no question he would receive it. In the last few years he's has two pulmonary embolisms, which are life-threatening blood clots. "The hospital treated him like a king," says his father. Like Bill, Evan is mainly non-verbal, can be hard to motivate, and needs help with showering and shaving. But he understands more than 90 per cent of what people say to him, laughs at all the right places at the movies, and curses appropriately. Evan will never be fully independent, so Ted has been saving up to ensure that, if Evan outlives him, "he'll have control over his lifestyle."[7]

Susan and Evan's parents worked to give their children the richest lives they could have. Mine did not. Part of the reason is a matter of simple definition. Susan and Evan are—and have always been—seen as individuals with a disability. Bill was, as my Dad put it, a Down syndrome youngster, not a youngster with Down syndrome. There's a world of difference between those two phrases. In my family, disability trumped everything, and Bill's world was so much the poorer for it.

Even so, Bill did have a chance to move into the larger world in the mid-1980s, when he was considered for a placement in Ottawa. He did not want to go, and my parents didn't want him to go either. Bill had no grounds for making his choice, however: all he knew was the institution. My parents did know, or could have known, or should have known about other possibilities. They could have consulted experts, talked to the families of other residents, sought advice on what would make it work for Bill. They could have asked Mary or Bob or me to help them learn more, or to do some research on the types of living arrangement that might be available. But they did not. They didn't even tell us it was a possibility. In the years between the time they sent Bill away and the time he could have left the institution, social attitudes toward disabilities had changed. Theirs had not.

And that's where I get angry. While I understand why they admitted him to the hospital school in the first place, I cannot understand why they left him there.

The Williston report, back in 1971, should have been a wakeup call. Bill's growing behavioural problems and declining language skills over the next few years should have been, too. The media coverage should have made our parents not just worry but think seriously about whether there was a better way for Bill to live. The hard work of the parents' groups fighting for integration should have given them hope and inspiration. Instead, they let their son be a permanent inmate at Rideau Regional. Down syndrome, for Bill, was a life sentence.

Mom said her biggest regret was that she and Dad didn't bring him home for visits. Mine is that I let them make all the decisions about Bill, even though I had less and less faith in their judgment as the years went by. I challenged them on a lot of things in life, including how I would raise my own children, but when it came to Bill I gave them a pass. I know that means I gave myself one, too. I let him be their son, their responsibility. In doing that, I became yet another in a long series of people who failed him.

He deserved better.

Acknowledgements

My brother's story has been a part of my life for almost as long as I can remember, but figuring out how to tell it was a long time coming. I had a lot of help along the way, and there are a number of people I want to thank.

Jim and Marilyn Dolmage and Vici Clarke, litigation guardians in the Huronia and Rideau Regional class-action suits, and David McKillop, the representative plaintiff in the Rideau Regional case, were incredibly patient and generous in answering my questions. So was Leah Dolmage, one of the driving forces behind the group working to rebuild the Huronia Cemetery. These people are heroes; without them the story of Ontario's shameful history of dealing with people with intellectual disabilities could easily have been forgotten. It was a privilege to speak with them.

I am deeply grateful to the dozen or so former staff members of Rideau Regional who shared their own experiences at the place, in interviews and through email. Some of them knew Bill and were able to round out my portrait of the brother who was an absence more than a presence in my family. Others offered honest and sometimes critical assessments of the promises and failures of the place. Though few are named in the book, their contributions to it are enormous.

Kate Rossiter of Wilfrid Laurier University in Brantford, Ontario, Judith Sandys of Ryerson University, and Victoria Freeman of York University shared their ideas, their stories, their work, and their resources with me. Janet Still and Ben Syposz made sure I had the details of Bill's medical condition right. My good friends and fellow writers Mary Somers, Norma Greenaway, and Erin Scullion encouraged me in this work and read drafts of the manuscript. Erin also put me in touch with her sister-in-law Bev, whose sister lived at the institution at the same time as my brother. The writers Stephen Kimber and Mark Bourrie offered helpful advice on how to get my story published. Marcel Rousseau very kindly shared a postcard image of Huronia from his private collection.

I'm grateful to the people at Goose Lane who saw the potential in this work, and especially to my editor, Jill Ainsley, who helped shape that potential into publishable form, and my copy editor, Kristen Chew, who improved my prose and saved me from many embarrassments.

I thank my friends for many hours of patient listening and gentle questioning as I tried to think my way to coherence on this story. I'm especially grateful to Jeanne Laux, Barbara Freeman, Carman Cumming, Debs Clark and many others for their kindness and support. Above all, I want to thank my family. My husband, Vincent Mosco, and my daughters, Rosemary and Madeline Mosco, have been in my corner from the beginning, as have my sister and brother, Mary and Bob McKercher. We all had our own experiences with Bill, and I am endlessly grateful to them for sharing theirs with me.

Researching the story of the institutions took me into unfamiliar areas of social policy, and sent me down many a rabbit hole of government documents. I have done my best to explain things fully and fairly. Any errors are, of course, my own. This book is mainly a work of history, examining the origin, rise, and fall of the institutional era in Ontario. The fact the institutions are closed is something to celebrate, but we still have a long way to go to live up to the principles set out by Walter Williston close to fifty years ago: "Society must provide each with such assistance, protection, opportunity and shelter as will enable him to take his place as a contributing member of the community and to ensure him a decent standard of living so that he can walk through life with dignity." My brother was robbed of that dignity. I hope his story will make us think about how to prevent that from happening to others like him, and remind us of how much more remains to be done.

Notes

Introduction "The **best thing** we could have done **for him**"

1. "Access to the Regional Centre Records," Ontario Ministry of Children, Community and Social Services, 2008, last modified Mar. 3, 2014, http://www.mcss.gov.on.ca/en/mcss/programs/developmental/huronia/index.aspx.

Chapter 1 "The great **Mongolian** family"

1. Elizabeth S. Stuart, *The Dalmeny Family of John and Jane McNabb Stuart/Stewart* (Osgoode, ON: published privately, 1997), 58.

2. Linda Robertson Paupst, *King Lineages and Memoirs* (Waterloo: Pendulum Press, 2003), 32.

3. "Attack Proves Fatal While Out Fishing," *North Bay Nugget*, Jun. 1934. See Paupst, *King Lineages*, 62.

4. My family always thought Bert volunteered, but his military record shows otherwise. See "Bertram McKercher," Personnel Records of the First World War, Library and Archives Canada, http://www.bac-lac.gc.ca/eng/discover/military-heritage/first-world-war/personnel-records/Pages/item.aspx?IdNumber=160645.

5. Dave Brown, "Trivial wartime tales amuse, and hide the scars," *Ottawa Citizen*, Oct. 4, 2010.

6. J. Langdon H. Down, "Observations on an Ethnic Classification of Idiots," *London Hospital Reports* 3, no. 1 (1866): 259–62, http://www.neonatology.org/classics/down.html.

7. Down, "Observations," 262.

8. "What is Down Syndrome?" US National Down Syndrome Society, https://www.ndss.org/about-down-syndrome/down-syndrome/. Trisomy 21

is the most common form of Down syndrome. Translocation, where the third copy of the chromosome 21 attaches itself to another chromosome, accounts for 4 per cent of cases. Mosaic Down syndrome, where some cells have 46 chromosomes and some have 47, is the rarest form and accounts for about 1 per cent.

9.   "Genes and Human Disease," Genomic Resource Centre, World Health Organization, http://www.who.int/genomics/public/geneticdiseases/en/; "Data and Statistics—Occurrence of Down Syndrome in the United States," US Centers for Disease Control, https://www.cdc.gov/ncbddd/birthdefects/downsyndrome/data.html; "Congenital Anomalies in Canada 2013: A Perinatal Health Surveillance Report," Public Health Agency of Canada, http://publications.gc.ca/site/eng/443924/publication.html; Gert de Graaf, Frank Buckley, and Brian G. Skotko, "Estimation of the number of people with Down syndrome in the United States," *Genetics in Medicine* 19, no. 4 (2017): 439-47, https://doi.org/10.1038/gim.2016.127.

10. "Data and Statistics," US Centers for Disease Control.

11. A.A. Diamandopoulos, K.G. Rakatsanis and N. Diamantopoulos, "A Neolithic Case of Down Syndrome?" *Journal of the History of the Neurosciences: Basic and Clinical Perspectives* 6, no. 1 (1997): 86–9.

12. Adam Hoffman, "New Fossils Hint 'Hobbit' Humans Are Older Than Thought," *National Geographic*, Jun. 8, 2016, https://news.nationalgeographic.com/2016/06/hobbits-humans-older-ancestors-island-fossils-archaeology/.

13. Down, "Observations."

14. David Wright, *Downs: The History of a Disability* (New York: Oxford University Press, 2011), 122.

15. A US Centers for Disease Control data sheet says that, as of 2007, the life expectancy for those with Down syndrome was 47; the Global Down Syndrome Foundation gives a life expectancy of 60. See "Data and Statistics," US Centers for Disease Control; "What is Down Syndrome?" US National Down Syndrome Society; the Global Down Syndrome Foundation, https://www.globaldownsyndrome.org/about-down-syndrome/facts-about-down-syndrome/.

16. Wright, *Downs*, 3.

17. Wright, *Downs*, 3.

18. Ann Gath, "The School-Aged Siblings of Mongol Children," *British Journal of Psychiatry* 123, no. 573 (1973): 161–7.

19. Created in 1956 to advise the provincial government on policy, this committee included representatives from more than a dozen social welfare agencies in Toronto. See "Interim Report—Committee on Needs of the Retarded," Dec. 23, 1957, Archives of Ontario, Regional Centre Records, CR118680.

Chapter 2 "A darling, **easy baby**"

1. "Top Names of the 1950s," US Social Security Administration, https://www.ssa.gov/OACT/babynames/decades/names1950s.html

2. Dorothy McKercher, personal letter, Dec. 1, 1985.

3. Peter L. Tyor and Leland V. Bell, *Caring for the Retarded in America: A History* (Westport, CT: Greenwood Press, 1984), x.

3. Tyor and Bell, *Caring for the Retarded in America*, x.

4. McKercher, personal letter.

5. Brian G. Skotko, "Gastrointestinal Tract and Down Syndrome," US National Down Syndrome Society, https://www.ndss.org/resources/gastrointestinal-tract-syndrome/.

6. McKercher, personal letter.

7. McKercher, personal letter.

8. McKercher, personal letter.

9. Brian G. Skotko and Susan P. Levine, "What the Other Children Are Thinking: Brothers and Sisters of Persons with Down Syndrome," *American Journal of Medical Genetics* 142, no. 3 (2006): 80–6.

10. Harvey G. Simmons, *From Asylum to Welfare* (Toronto: National Institute on Mental Retardation, 1982), 151.

11. Doug McKercher, letter to Harold Frank, Oct. 9, 1958.

Chapter 3 "Hospitals for **mental defectives**"

1. E.M. Itard, *An Historical Account of the Development and Education of A Savage Man* (London: Richard Philips, 1802), 14.

2. Jonathan Plucker, "Jean-Marc Gaspard Itard," Human Intelligence: Historical Influences, Current Controversies, Teaching Resources (web site), last modified Apr. 28, 2018, https://www.intelltheory.com/itard.shtml.

3. Peter L. Tyor and Leland V. Bell, *Caring for the Retarded in America: A History* (Westport, CT: Greenwood Press, 1984), 15.

4. David Wright, *Downs: The History of a Disability* (New York: Oxford University Press, 2011), 41.

5. Penny L. Richards, "Beside Her Sat Her Idiot Child: Families and Developmental Disability in Mid-Nineteenth-Century America," in *Mental Retardation in America: A Historical Reader*, ed. Steven Noll and James W. Trent (New York: NYU Press, 2004), 70.

6. Tyor and Bell, *Caring for the Retarded in America*, 15.

7. Tyor and Bell, *Caring for the Retarded in America*, 25.

8. Tyor and Bell, *Caring for the Retarded in America*, xi.

9. Deborah Cohen, *Family Secrets: Shame and Privacy in Modern Britain* (Oxford: Oxford University Press, 2013), 90.

10. J. Langdon H. Down, "Observations on an Ethnic Classification of Idiots," *London Hospital Reports* 3, no. 1 (1866): 259–62.

11. Down, "Observations," 260–61.

12. An image of the original Normansfield advertisement and a history of the institution can be found at the Langdon Down Museum of Learning Disability. See https://langdondownmuseum.org.uk/dr-john-langdon-down/normansfield/.

13. "Normansfield," Langdon Down Museum of Learning Disability, https://langdondownmuseum.org.uk/dr-john-langdon-down/normansfield/.

14. Cohen, *Family Secrets,* 94.

15. Cohen, *Family Secrets,* 87.

16. Cohen, *Family Secrets,* 90.

17. Harvey G. Simmons, *From Asylum to Welfare* (Toronto: National Institute on Mental Retardation, 1982), 5.

18. Simmons, *From Asylum to Welfare,* 25–56.

19. Kate Rossiter and Annalise Clarkson, "Opening Ontario's 'Saddest Chapter': A Social History of Huronia Regional Centre," *Canadian Journal of Disability Studies* 2, no. 3 (2013): 5.

20. Simmons, *From Asylum to Welfare,* 37–41.

21. Simmons, *From Asylum to Welfare,* 39.

22. Tyor and Bell, *Caring for the Retarded in America*, 36.

23. Tyor and Bell, *Caring for the Retarded in America*, 38.

24. Tyor and Bell, *Caring for the Retarded in America*, 70.

25. Tyor and Bell, *Caring for the Retarded in America*, 34.

26. Pauline Morris, *Put Away: A Sociological Study of Institutions for the Mentally Retarded* (London: Routledge and Kegan Paul, 1969), 10.

27. Cohen, *Family Secrets*, 108.

28. Morris, *Put Away*, 10.

29. Cohen, *Family Secrets*, 107–108.

30. Cohen, *Family Secrets*, 89. Reginald also added a hyphen to his surname.

31. The province asked MacMurchy to conduct a census of the feeble-minded in 1905 and, as Simmons writes, "From that point on her reports on the feeble-minded appeared in the Ontario Sessional Papers." Initially, MacMurchy worked without a formal title but, in 1914, she was appointed Inspector of the Feeble-Minded (Simmons, *From Asylum to Welfare*, 67).

32. Don Butler, "The dark side of honouring Dr. Helen MacMurchy," *Ottawa Citizen*, May 5, 2012.

33. Simmons, *From Asylum to Welfare*, 132.

34. DeNeen L. Brown, "Civil rights crusader Fannie Lou Hamer defied men—and presidents—who tried to silence her," *Washington Post*, Oct. 6, 2017.

35. Roger Collier, "Reports of Coerced Sterilization of Indigenous Women in Canada Mirrors Shameful Past," *Canadian Medical Association Journal*, Aug. 2, 2017, https://cmajnews.com/2017/08/02/reports-of-coerced-sterilization-of-indigenous-women-in-canada-mirrors-shameful-past-cmaj-109-5471/. Collier notes that forced sterilization of Indigenous women was supposed to have ended in the 1970s, but reports of Indigenous women being coerced into having their tubes tied, often while they are in labour, continue to this day.

36. Cohen, *Family Secrets*, 115 and 116.

37. James. W. Trent, *Inventing the Feeble Mind: A History of Mental Retardation in the United States* (Berkeley and Los Angeles: University of California Press, 1994), 187.

38. Simmons, *From Asylum to Welfare*, 134.

39. Thelma Wheatley, *"And Neither Have I Wings to Fly"— Labelled and Locked Up in an Institution* (Toronto: Inanna Publications, 2013).

40. "New Provincial hospital may be located here," *Smiths Falls Record News*, May 17, 1934; "No Announcement of Hospital but Work Proceeding Rapidly," *Smiths Falls Record News*, May 24, 1934.

41. "Minister of Health Makes Announcement of Hospital," *Smiths Falls Record News*, Jun. 14, 1934.

42. "Public accounts of the province of Ontario for the year ended Oct. 31 1934," Government of Ontario (Toronto: T.E. Bowman), https://archive.org/details/publicaccounts1934onta; "Public accounts of the province of Ontario for the year ended Mar. 31 1935," Government of Ontario (Toronto: T.E. Bowman), https://archive.org/details/publicaccounts1935onta.

43. "Open Way to Hospital," *Smiths Falls Record News*, Jul. 18, 1946.

44. "Doucet announced hospital for Smiths Falls," *Smiths Falls Record News*, Aug. 22, 1946.

45. Walter B. Williston, *Present Arrangements for the Care and Supervision of Mentally Retarded Persons in Ontario* (Toronto: Ontario Department of Health, 1971), 37.

46. Wolf Wolfensberger, "Models of Mental Retardation," *New Society* 15 (1970): 51–3. Reprinted in *Leadership and Change in Human Services: Selected Readings from Wolf Wolfensberger*, ed. David G. Race (London: Routledge, 2003), 19.

Chapter 4 "Progress and happiness"

1. Glenn J. Lockwood, *Smiths Falls: A Social History of the Men and Women in a Rideau Canal Community 1794-1994* (Smiths Falls: Heritage House Museum, 1994), 509.

2. "Facts and Figures: Working at the Rideau Regional Centre," *Rideau Regional Centre Memory Book 1951-2001*, History of Developmental Services, Ontario Ministry of Community and Social Services, last modified Mar. 8, 2018, http://www.mcss.gov.on.ca/en/dshistory/working/facts_figures.aspx.

3. Sue Ronald, "Rideau Regional Centre 1951-1986: A History of Serving the Handicapped," *Rideau Regional Centre Celebrates 35 Years of Helping the Handicapped*. Commemorative booklet, 1986.

4. Memo from H.F. Frank, Medical Superintendent, Ontario Hospital School Smiths Falls, to Dr. B.H. McNeel, Chief, Medical Health Division, Ontario Department of Health, May 15, 1958, Archives of Ontario, Regional Centre Records, RCR010741.

5. "Rideau Regional Centre," History of Developmental Services, Ontario Ministry of Community and Social Services, http://www.mcss.gov.on.ca/en/dshistory/firstInstitution/rideau.aspx; Marvin Schiff, "Hospital School for Retarded Branded a Curse," *Globe and Mail*, Jan. 29, 1965.

6. Wolf Wolfensberger, "Models of Mental Retardation," *New Society* 15 (1970): 51–3. Reprinted in *Leadership and Change in Human Services: Selected Readings from Wolf Wolfensberger*, ed. David G. Race (London: Routledge, 2003), 51–3.

7. R.A. Farmer, "A historical cohort study to investigate the possible association between the use of depomedroxyprogesterone acetate (DMPA or Depo-Provera) and breast cancer in a population of institutionalized mentally retarded women," Operational Support Branch, Ministry of Community and Social Services, Dec. 1985, 28, Archives of Ontario, Rideau Regional Records, CR160287.

8. Donald E. Zarfas, Ian Fyfe, and Fabian Gorodzinsky, "The utilization of Depo-Provera in the Ontario government facilities for the mentally retarded: A pilot project," Oct. 1981, 9–10, Archives of Ontario, Rideau Regional Records, RCR002836.

9. "Viewpoint: Retarded resident writes," *Smiths Falls Record News*, Feb. 3, 1972.

10. *One on Every Street*, directed by George Gorman (Ontario: Department of Health/Fletcher Film Production, 1960), DVD.

11. *Danny and Nicky*, directed by Douglas Jackson (Canada: National Film Board of Canada, 1969), DVD.

12. Erving Goffman, *Asylums: Essays on the Social Situation of Mental Patients and Other Inmates* (New York: Doubleday, 1961).

Chapter 5 "Little, well nourished Mongolian"

1. Glenn J. Lockwood, *Smiths Falls: A Social History of the Men and Women in a Rideau Canal Community 1794-1994* (Smiths Falls: Heritage House Museum, 1994), 510. J.A. Gallipeau, which bought the property in 2011 for $100,000, with plans to turn it into housing for seniors, used the term in promotional material. See "Gallipeau Centre, Wood Mausoleum part of Doors Open event," *Smiths Falls Record News*, May 17, 2012.

2. David McKillop, interview with author, Jul. 11, 2018.

3. Sandy Baker Lennox, interview with author, May 9, 2018.

Chapter 6 "Very institutionalized"

1. "IQ Classifications in Educational Use," Assessment Psychology Online, last updated Jul. 17, 2016, http://www.assessmentpsychology.com/iqclassifications.htm. These terms went out of use in the 1970s.

2. "Ward Schooling," History of Developmental Services, Ontario Ministry of Community and Social Services, https://www.mcss.gov.on.ca/en/dshistory/lifeInstitution/ward_schooling.aspx.

3. "Trichotillomania (Hair Pulling)," Mental Health America, http://www.mentalhealthamerica.net/conditions/trichotillomania-hair-pulling.

4. "Trichotillomania (Hair-Pulling Disorder)," Mayo Clinic, http://www.mayoclinic.org/diseases-conditions/trichotillomania/symptoms-causes/dxc-20268523.

5. "Mental Health Issues and Down Syndrome," National Down Syndrome Society, https://www.ndss.org/resources/mental-health-issues-syndrome/.

6. Marvin Schiff, "Hospital School for Retarded Branded a Curse," *Globe and Mail*, Jan. 29, 1965.

Chapter 7 "A century of **failure** and **inhumanity**"

1. James. W. Trent, *Inventing the Feeble Mind: A History of Mental Retardation in the United States* (Berkeley and Los Angeles: University of California Press, 1994), 240.

2. "History," Canadian Association for Community Living, https://cacl.ca/who-we-are/about-us/. The name of the national group has changed several times over the years, reflecting both the changing nature of its work and changing attitudes in society. In 1969 it became the Canadian Association for the Mentally Retarded, to recognize that children grow up and still face discrimination and exclusion. In 1985 it became the Canadian Association for Community Living, focusing on creating communities emphasizing equality and diversity.

3. Like the national association, the Ontario group has also changed its name. It is now known as Community Living Ontario.

4. Harvey G. Simmons, *From Asylum to Welfare* (Toronto: National Institute on Mental Retardation, 1982), 149.

5. Simmons, *From Asylum to Welfare*, 149.

6. Simmons, *From Asylum to Welfare*, 149.

7. Betty Anglin and June Braaten, *Twenty-five Years of Growing Together: A History of the Ontario Association for the Mentally Retarded* (Toronto: Canadian Association for the Mentally Retarded, 1978), 11.

8. Anglin and Braaten, *Twenty-five Years*, 13.

9. Simmons, *From Asylum to Welfare*, 152.

10. "John F. Kennedy and People with Intellectual Disabilities," John F. Kennedy Presidential Library and Museum, https://www.jfklibrary.org/JFK/JFK-in-History/JFK-and-People-with-Intellectual-Disabilities.aspx.

11. Anglin and Braaten, *Twenty-five Years*, 36.

12. Simmons, *From Asylum to Welfare*, 195.

13. Simmons, *From Asylum to Welfare*, 185.

14. Simmons, *From Asylum to Welfare*, 185.

15. Trent, *Inventing the Feeble Mind*, 226.

16. David J. Rothman and Sheila M. Rothman, *The Willowbrook Wars: Bringing the Mentally Disabled Into the Community* (New Brunswick, NJ: AldineTransaction, 2005), 23.

17. Geraldo Rivera, "The last great disgrace," *Eyewitness News*, 1972, http://index.geraldo.com/page/willowbrook.

18. Pierre Berton, "What's wrong at Orillia: Out of sight, out of mind," *Toronto Star*, Jan. 6, 1960; republished as "Huronia: Pierre Berton warned us 50 years ago," *Toronto Star*, Sept. 20, 2013.

19. A.B. McKillop, *Pierre Berton: A Biography* (Toronto: McClelland and Stewart, 2008), 344–45.

20. Marvin Schiff, "Hospital School for Retarded Branded a Curse," *Globe and Mail*, Jan. 29, 1965.

21. "Parents of hurt boy ask hospital schools probe," *Globe and Mail*, Oct. 28 1966.

22. "Lewis says crowding hospital death cause," *Globe and Mail*, Feb. 16, 1967.

23. "Dog finds children," *Globe and Mail*, Apr. 15, 1969.

24. The accounts of Sanderson's death and Martel's injuries are drawn from Walter B. Williston, *Present Arrangements for the Special Care and Supervision of Mentally Retarded Persons in Ontario*, report to the Ontario Minister of Health, Aug. 1971, 8–19.

25. Williston, *Present Arrangements*, 4–5.

26. Williston, *Present Arrangements*, 68.

27. Williston, *Present Arrangements*, 8.

28. Williston, *Present Arrangements*, 36–38.

29. Williston, *Present Arrangements*, 38.

30. Williston, *Present Arrangements*, 40–41.

31. Williston, *Present Arrangements*, 39.

32. Williston, *Present Arrangements*, 39.

33. Williston, *Present Arrangements*, 66.

34. Williston, *Present Arrangements*, 67.

35. Williston, *Present Arrangements*, 69.

36. Williston, *Present Arrangements*, 73–83.

37. Edna Hampton, "Lawrence promises care for retarded within community in five years," *Globe and Mail*, Sept. 17, 1971.

38. Wolf Wolfensberger, "Mental retardation," letter to the editor, *Globe and Mail*, Nov. 1, 1971, 6.

39. Simmons, *From Asylum to Welfare*, 203.

40 Robert Welch, *Community Living for the Mentally Retarded in Ontario: A New Policy Focus* (Toronto: Cabinet Committee on Social Development, Mar. 1973), 1.

41. Simmons, *From Asylum to Welfare*, 207.

42. Anglin and Braaten, *Twenty-five Years*, 70.

Chapter 8 "Only when he becomes more **advanced"**

1. "Study Details Development of Functional Skills in Persons with Down Syndrome," Massachusetts General Hospital, Jan. 2, 2019, https://www. newswise.com/articles/study-details-development-of-functional-skills-in-persons-with-down-syndrome.

2. Barbara Yaffe, "Residents of homes for retarded drugged to keep them docile," *Globe and Mail*, May 5, 1977.

3. Barbara Yaffe, "Controversial treatment for profoundly retarded," *Globe and Mail*, Mar. 3, 1977.

4. "Interim guidelines for the use of behavior modification," undated memo, Archives of Ontario, Rideau Regional Records, RCR009083.

5. "Obsessive Compulsive Behavior—Overview," Mayo Clinic, http://www. mayoclinic.org/diseases-conditions/obsessive-compulsive-disorder/home/ ovc-20245947.

6. "Obsessive Compulsive Behavior," *Psychology Today*, last updated Mar. 5, 2018, https://www.psychologytoday.com/conditions/ obsessive-compulsive-disorder.

7. "Facts and Statistics," Anxiety and Depression Association of America, https://adaa.org/about-adaa/press-room/facts-statistics; "Mental Health

Issues & Down syndrome," National Down syndrome Society, https://www.ndss.org/resources/mental-health-issues-syndrome/.

8. For a discussion of current issues around group homes, see Natalie Spagnuolo, "Building Back Wards in a (Post) Institutional Era: Hospital Confinement, Group Home Eviction and Ontario's Treatment of People Labeled with Intellectual Difficulties," *Disability Studies Quarterly* 36, no. 4 (2016), http://dsq-sds.org/article/view/5279/4480.

9. Andy Shanks, interview with author, Jun. 3, 2018.

10. Sandy Baker Lennox, interview with author, May 9, 2018.

Chapter 9 "Inclusion, independence and choice"

1. Ivan Brown and John P. Radford, "The Growth and Decline of Institutions for People with Developmental Disabilities in Ontario: 1876-2009," *Journal on Developmental Disabilities* 21, no. 2 (2015): 24.

2. "The Shift to Community Living," History of Developmental Services, Ontario Ministry of Community and Social Services, http://www.mcss.gov.on.ca/en/dshistory/community/index.aspx.

3. The report, "COMSOC, Transfer of Mental Retardation Services: Proposals for a Transfer Timetable," came from the firm Hickling-Johnston in August 1973. See Harvey G. Simmons, *From Asylum to Welfare* (Toronto: National Institute on Mental Retardation, 1982), 209–10.

4. Three Schedule 1 institutions were "delisted" in 1974 under the Developmental Services Act and five more were opened between 1974 and 1976. "Government-Operated Institutions for People with a Developmental Disability," History of Developmental Services, Ministry of Children, Community and Social Services, https://www.mcss.gov.on.ca/en/dshistory/firstInstitution/list_institutions.aspx.

5. "How Justin Clark's fight for independence transformed disability rights in Canada," CBC, *The Sunday Edition*, Nov. 25, 2018, https://www.cbc.ca/radio/thesundayedition/november-25-2018-the-sunday-edition-with-michael-enright-1.4911588/how-justin-clark-s-fight-for-independence-transformed-disability-rights-in-canada-1.4911590.

6. Simmons, *From Asylum to Welfare*, 216.

7. Kathleen Rex, "Taylor fears backlash if retarded moved home too fast," *Globe and Mail*, Apr. 23, 1976.

8. "Group home stands empty in Etobicoke: Zoning slows plan to move retarded into community," *Globe and Mail*, Nov. 11, 1976.

9. Kevin Marron, "The Catch-22 of Group Home Bylaws," *Canadian Lawyer*, May 12, 2012, https://www.canadianlawyermag.com/author/kevin-marron/the-catch-22-of-group-home-bylaws-1596/.

10. Oliver Moore, "Community applauds Doug Ford's opposition of youth group home," *Globe and Mail*, May 18, 2014.

11. Laurie Monsebraaten, "Councillor Doug Ford's group home comments shock and sadden Autism advocates," *Toronto Star*, May 20, 2014.

12. Memo marked "confidential" from Robert Welch, provincial secretary for social development, to W. Darcy McKeough, MPP, Apr. 25, 1973, Archives of Ontario, Regional Centre Records, RCR026508.

13. Stan Oziewicz, "Retarded children sterilized illegally, guardian contends," *Globe and Mail*, Dec. 12, 1978.

14. "Sterilization and hysterectomies performed on residents in Schedule 1 M.R. facilities in Ontario (government operated) from 1970-1976," undated spreadsheet, Archives of Ontario, Regional Centre Records, CR033586; "Contentious issue: sterilization," Briefing note, Dec. 12, 1978, Archives of Ontario, Regional Centre Records, RCR032595.

15. "500 retarded sterilized, Quebec reports," *Globe and Mail*, Jul. 3, 1980.

16. "Psychiatrists condemn practice of letting retarded babies die," *Globe and Mail*, Feb. 16, 1979.

17. Simmons, *From Asylum to Welfare*, 218–19.

18. Betty Anglin and June Braaten, *Twenty-five Years of Growing Together: A History of the Ontario Association for the Mentally Retarded* (Toronto: Canadian Association for the Mentally Retarded, 1978), 70.

19. Rosemarie Boyle, "From dreary wards to life's backwaters," *Globe and Mail*, Feb. 12, 1976.

20. Simmons, *From Asylum to Welfare*, 236.

21. Simmons, *From Asylum to Welfare*, 237.

22. Paul Knox, "End sought to double standard for retarded," *Globe and Mail*, Mar. 17, 1980, 5.

23. Beverly Scullion, interview with author, Jun. 6, 2018.

24. Frank Drea, update on new five-year plan, *Debates of the Legislative Assembly of Ontario*, Apr. 28, 1983.

25. Drea, update, *Debates*, Apr. 28, 1983.

26. Bruce McCaffrey, response to questions, *Debates of the Legislative Assembly of Ontario*, Oct. 18, 1983.

27. *Challenges and Opportunities: Community Living for People with Developmental Handicaps*, Ontario Ministry of Community and Social Services, May 1987.

28. "Challenges and Opportunities," 6–8.

29. Canadian Centre for Policy Alternatives, "The Long Shadow of Mike Harris," *On Policy* (Summer 2015), www.policyalternatives.ca/publications/reports/onpolicy-long-shadow-mike-harris.

30. Stephen Anderson and Sonia Ben Jaafar, "Policy Trends in Ontario Education 1990-2003," Ontario Institute for Studies in Education (OISE), University of Toronto, Sept. 2003, http://fcis.oise.utoronto.ca/~icec/policytrends.pdf.

31. "Making Services Work for People," Ministry of Community and Social Services, Apr. 1997, http://www.ontla.on.ca/library/repository/mon/1000/10264783.pdf.

32. Ottawa-Carleton Association for Persons with Developmental Disabilities, "A Timeline," https://www.ocapdd.on.ca/?ID=84&Language=ENG.

33. "Disabled people to get more funds," *Globe and Mail*, May 6, 2000.

34. Tom Blackwell, "Ontario could close institutions for mentally disabled," *National Post*, Sept. 15, 2000.

35. Don Gallant, interview with author, Jul. 16, 2018.

36. "Newfoundland and Labrador," provincial and territorial updates, InstitutionWatch.ca, Oct. 5, 2007, http://www.institutionwatch.ca/iwupdates-app/prov.Newfoundland%20and%20Labrador (page discontinued).

37. L'Arche Canada, *A resource document on Institutions and De-Institutionalization*, for the Ontario "Canadian and World Studies" curriculum, 2014, 13–14; Rob Shaw, "B.C. government to compensate pre-1974 Woodlands residents," *Province*, Mar, 30, 2018, updated Mar. 31, 2018.

38. Laura Glowacki, "$50M lawsuit alleges intellectually disabled residents were sexually abused, starved at Manitoba institution," CBC, Dec. 19, 2018, https://www.cbc.ca/news/canada/manitoba/manitoba-developmental-centre-class-action-1.4898001; Arthur White-Crummey, "Class action over alleged abuse at Valley View Centre back before courts," *Regina Leader-Post*, Sept. 14, 2018.

39. European Intellectual Disability Network, *Intellectual Disability in Europe: Working Papers* (Canterbury: Tizard Centre, University of Kent at Canterbury, 2003), http://www.enil.eu/wp-content/uploads/2012/07/

Intellectual-Disability-in-Europe.pdf; Eric Lipton, "Move to close Va. institutions for the retarded concerns some parents," *Washington Post*, Mar. 11, 1996; Raymond A. Lemay, "Deinstitutionalization of People With Developmental Disabilities: A Review of the Literature," *Canadian Journal of Community Mental Health*, 28, no. 1 (2009): 181–94.

40. Disability Justice Resource Centre, "The Closing of Willowbrook," http://disabilityjustice.org/the-closing-of-willowbrook/; David J. Rothman and Sheila M. Rothman, *The Willowbrook Wars: Bringing the Mentally Disabled Into the Community* (New Brunswick, NJ: AldineTransaction, 2005); David Levine, "The Real History of Letchworth Village," *Hudson Valley Magazine*, Feb. 2, 2016.

41. "The Normansfield Inquiry," *British Medical Journal* 2, no. 6151 (1978), 1560–63; Terry Philpot, "Museum opens door to hospital's past," *Guardian*, Feb. 2, 2012.

42. Richard Mackie and Margaret Philp, "Developmental disability homes to be closed," *Globe and Mail*, Sept. 10, 2004.

43. "Numbers of persons reported in mental retardation survey III (May 31 1972) by mental retardation facility and age," Jan. 15, 1973, Archives of Ontario, Regional Centre Records, RCR022990; "Planning for the closure of DS facilities and placement of clients," confidential draft for discussion by the Program Management Committee, Oct. 15, 2003, Archives of Ontario, Regional Centre Records, CR162120.

44. Norman W. Sterling, *Debates of the Legislative Assembly of Ontario*, Oct. 19, 2004.

45. "Closure of developmental service facilities 'heartless,' says union," news release, Sept. 9, 2004, Archives of Ontario, Regional Centre Records, HRCE027428.

46. Norman W. Sterling, *Debates of the Legislative Assembly of Ontario*, Apr. 4 and Nov. 30, 2005, and Mar. 21, 2007.

47. Ian Sutton, "Group homes row goes to court," *Globe and Mail*, Dec. 12, 2015.

48. Ian Sutton, "Court decision seen as victory for developmentally disabled," *Globe and Mail*, Jan. 27, 2006.

49. Dorothy Griffiths, Frances Owen, and Rosemary Condillac, *Facilities Initiative: Final Case Studies Report* (Centre for Applied Disability Studies, Brock University, 2012), 84–166.

50. Dorothy Griffiths, Frances Owen, and Rosemary Condillac, *Final Report of Agency and Family Surveys* (Centre for Applied Disability Studies, Brock University, 2010), 6.

51. Griffiths, Owen, and Condillac, *Final Report*, 7–30.

52. Andrew Duffy, "Closing of Rideau Regional Centre to be 'historic day'; Institute once home to more than 2,500 developmentally disabled people," *Ottawa Citizen*, Mar. 13, 2009.

53. "Residents, staff mark closure of Rideau Regional Centre," *St. Lawrence EMC*, Apr. 2, 2009.

Chapter 10 "Red flagged"

1. Walter M. Robinson and Brandon T. Unruh, "The Hepatitis Experiments at Willowbrook State School," in *The Oxford Textbook of Clinical Research Ethics*, ed. Ezekiel J. Emanuel et al. (New York: Oxford University Press, 2008), 80–85; Saul Krugman, "The Willowbrook Hepatitis Studies Revisited: Ethical Aspects," *Reviews of Infectious Diseases* 8, no. 1 (1986): 157–62.

2. "Acute vs. Chronic Infection," The Hepatitis B Foundation, http://www.hepb.org/what-is-hepatitis-b/what-is-hepb/acute-vs-chronic/; "Hepatitis B—Key Facts," World Health Organization, last updated Jul. 18, 2018, http://www.who.int/news-room/fact-sheets/detail/hepatitis-b.

3. "Hepatitis project 1975," memo by E. Perry, Department Of Microbiology and Immunology, University of Ottawa, Jan. 21, 1975, Archives of Ontario, Regional Centre Records, CR118305; R.K. Chaudhary et al., letter to the editor, *The New England Journal of Medicine* 327, no. 27 (Dec. 31, 1992).

4. Michael A. Kerr, "The Immune System in Down's Syndrome," Intellectual Disability and Health, University of Hertfordshire, http://www.intellectualdisability.info/physical-health/articles/the-immune-system-in-downs-syndrome.

5. "Infectious hepatitis—Ontario Hospital School, Smiths Falls," undated report, Archives of Ontario, Regional Centre Records, RCR023548.

6. "Infectious hepatitis—Ontario Hospital School, Smiths Falls," RCR023548.

7. "Infectious hepatitis, Ontario Hospital School, Smiths Falls," Feb. 26, 1962, Archives of Ontario, Regional Centre Records, RCR023515. An earlier version of this memo is marked "rough draft" RCR023507.

8. "O.H.S. Smiths Falls visit Apr. 24-29, 1962," typed and handwritten notes, Archives of Ontario, Regional Centre Records, RCR023585.

9. Dr. N. Lysander, Administrator, Rideau Regional Centre, "Policy memo 160," Feb. 28, 1978, Archives of Ontario, Regional Centre Records, RCR045368.

10. "Why People with Down Syndrome Invariably Develop Alzheimer's Disease," *NeuroscienceNews.com*, Oct. 23, 2014, http://neurosciencenews.com/snx27-beta-amyloid-down-syndrome-1470/.

11. Ann Gedye, *Dementia Scale for Down Syndrome* (Vancouver: Gedye Research and Consulting, 1995).

12. As I mentioned in the Introduction, I agreed not to reveal the names of people named in the database at the Archives of Ontario as a condition of access. I have taken the same approach with Bill's file.

Chapter 11 "An air of **violence** and **punishment**"

1. Beth Marlin, "A chance for Huronia's 'invisible' to be seen and heard," *Globe and Mail*, Jul. 26, 2010.

2. Carol Goar, "The hidden heroes of Huronia," *Toronto Star*, Sept. 29, 2013.

3. Class certification order between Marilyn Dolmage as litigation guardian of Marie Slark and Jim Dolmage as litigation guardian of Patricia Seth and Her Majesty the Queen in right of the Province of Ontario and Huronia Regional Centre, Ontario Superior Court of Justice, Toronto, Jul. 30, 2010; court file number CV-09-378927CP00.

4. The Rideau Regional claim launched in September 2010 and the Southwestern Ontario at the end of December that year. Both classes used the same legal firm as the Huronia suit, and both were certified on August 19, 2011.

5. Huronia statement of claim between Marilyn Dolmage as litigation guardian of Marie Slark and Jim Dolmage as litigation guardian of Patricia Seth and Her Majesty the Queen in right of the Province of Ontario and Huronia Regional Centre, Ontario Superior Court of Justice, Toronto, Apr. 21, 2009, 11.

6. Huronia claim, 11–12.

7. Rideau Regional statement of claim between David McKillop by his litigation guardian Christine Victoria Grace Clarke and her Majesty the Queen in right of the Province of Ontario, Ontario Superior Court of Justice, Toronto, Sept. 24, 2010, 9.

8. Southwestern Ontario statement of claim between Rosalind Bechard as litigation guardian of Mary Ellen Fox and Her Majesty the Queen in right of the Province of Ontario, Ontario Superior Court of Justice, Toronto, Dec. 29, 2010, 9–10.

9. In an interview Jul. 11, 2018, he told me they were too small and too tight and permanently damaged his feet.

10. Rideau Regional claim, 9.

11. Rideau Regional claim, 9.

12. Rideau Regional claim, 16.

13. Rideau Regional claim, 18–19.

14. Huronia statement of defence, Marilyn Dolmage as litigation guardian of Marie Slark and Jim Dolmage as litigation guardian of Patricia Seth versus Her Majesty the Queen in right of the Province of Ontario and Huronia Regional Centre, Ontario Superior Court of Justice, Toronto, Jan. 31, 2011, 11.

15. Huronia statement of defence, 6.

16. Huronia statement of defence, 14.

17. Huronia statement of defence, 12.

18. Rachel Mendleson, "Huronia lawsuit against Ontario government delayed without explanation," *Toronto Star*, Sept. 16, 2013.

19. Marilyn and Jim Dolmage, interview with author, Apr. 12, 2018.

20. Paola Loriggio, "Huronia Regional Centre Lawsuit: $35-Million Settlement In Class-Action Suit Over Alleged Abuse," *Canadian Press*, Sept. 17, 2013.

21. Rachel Mendleson, "Huronia institution cemetery a painful reminder of neglect and abuse," *Toronto Star*, Sept. 17, 2013.

22. Mendleson, "Huronia institution cemetery"; see also Tim Alamenciak, "Remembering the dead at Huronia Regional Centre," *Toronto Star*, Dec. 29, 2014.

23. Kathleen Wynne, *Debates of the Legislative Assembly of Ontario*, Dec. 9, 2013.

24. "Two more settlements reached over alleged abuse at Ontario institutions," *Canadian Press*, Dec. 24, 2013.

25. "Premier Kathleen Wynne's apology to Huronia survivors offers fresh start," *Toronto Star*, Dec. 9, 2013.

26. Tim Alamenciak, "Huronia: Settled but not forgotten," *Toronto Star*, Sept. 30, 2013.

27. Marco Chown Oved, "Group says it found a sewage pipe in Huronia cemetery," *Toronto Star*, Jul. 31, 2015.

28. Leah Dolmage, interview with author, Apr. 16, 2018.

29. Tim Alamenciak, "Huronia survivors told some case files are missing," *Toronto Star*, Jul. 6, 2014.

30. Marilyn Dolmage, interview with author, Apr. 23, 2018.

31. Settlement and legal fees approval, Sharon Clegg as Litigation Guardian of Marlene McIntyre, Representative Plaintiff of Certified Class Action, and Her Majesty the Queen in Right of the Province of Ontario, defendant, Ontario Superior Court, Apr. 28, 2018, 7.

32. "Settlement Reached in Developmental Facilities Class Action," Government of Ontario, archived news release, Apr. 27, 2016; Michelle McQuigge, "Class action over alleged abuse at Ontario school for the blind ends in $8-million settlement," *Toronto Star*, Apr. 8, 2017.

33. Paola Loriggio, "Lawsuit filed by Timmins family alleges people with developmental disabilities denied necessary services," *Canadian Press*, Apr. 24, 2017.

34. Alex Ballingall, "Former Huronia residents join speakers' series to educate others on horrors endured," *Toronto Star*, Feb. 10, 2016.

35. Kate Rossiter and Jen Rinaldi, *Institutional Violence and Disability: Punishing Conditions* (London: Routledge: 2019).

36. Muriel Draaisma, "Institutions are breeding grounds for violence, Laurier prof argues in new book," CBC News, Kitchener-Waterloo, Aug 23, 2018, https://www.cbc.ca/news/canada/kitchener-waterloo/institutional-violence-huronia-regional-centre-laurier-professor-1.4796117.

37. Huronia statement of defence, Jan. 31, 2011, 18.

38. Keith Norton, response to Mr. Blundy, Mar. 17, 1979, Archives of Ontario, Regional Centre Records, CR009563.

39. The reports I describe in this section contain names, dates, locations, and other identifying information. To comply with the research agreement, I have summarized the contents and have chosen to not cite the document numbers.

40. Stacey Roy, "Former Rideau staff seek premier's apology through online petition," *Smiths Falls Record News*, Jan. 22, 2015.

41. See, for example, Madeline C. Burghardt, *Broken: Institutions, Families and the Construction of Intellectual Disability* (Montreal and Kingston: McGill-Queen's Press, 2019).

Chapter 12 "We never seem to **find time** to **talk about Bill**"

1. Elizabeth S. Stuart, *The Dalmeny Family of John and Jane McNabb Stuart/Stewart* (Osgoode, ON: published privately, 1997), 91.

2. George F. Will, "The real Down syndrome problem: Accepting genocide," *Washington Post*, Mar. 14, 2018.

3. Michael Berube, "This Pa. abortion bill has nothing to do with helping kids with Down syndrome or their families," PennLive.com, updated Apr. 6, 2018, http://www.pennlive.com/opinion/2018/04/this_pa_abortion_bill_has_noth.html.

4. Robert Munsch, *Love You Forever* (Richmond Hill, ON: Firefly Books, 1995).

5. David Wright, *Downs: The History of a Disability* (New York: Oxford University Press, 2011), 4.

6. Wright, *Downs*, 6.

7. Interview with author, Aug. 4, 2018.

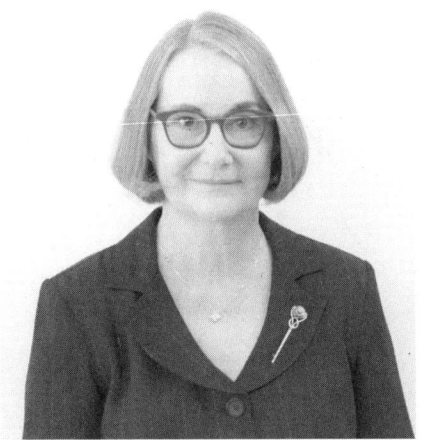

Catherine McKercher worked as a journalist for the *Ottawa Journal*, the Canadian Press (serving as a correspondent in Toronto and Washington), and the *Kingston Whig-Standard* before becoming a professor of journalism at Carleton University, where she taught for 27 years. She has written and edited a number of books, including *Newsworkers Unite: Labor, Convergence and North American Newspapers*, a history of newspaper labour unions in the information age; *The Canadian Reporter: News Writing and Reporting*, a leading journalism textbook co-authored with Carleton colleagues that is in its third edition; and a pair of volumes with Vincent Mosco, *Knowledge Workers in the Information Society* and *The Laboring of Communication*. Catherine McKercher is Professor Emerita at Carleton University.